THE CARCINOID SYNDROME SURVIVOR GUIDE

Transform Your Health and Discover Nourishing Recipes for Symptoms Alleviation and Relief

Michael Slowick, RDN

COPYRIGHT PAGE

to ensure the accuracy of the information provided herein, no promises are made regarding its completeness or accuracy. Any statements made by sales employees or representatives, whether verbal or written, do not constitute extended or implied guarantees.

Table of Contents

COPYRIGHT PAGE.. 2

Table of Contents 4

INTRODUCTION 1

CHAPTER I: WHAT EXACTLY IS CARCINOID SYNDROME?.. 3

Causes of Cardiovascular Syndrome...................... 6

Indications of Cardinod Syndrome........................ 14

CHAPTER II: DIAGNOSIS OF CARCINOID SYNDROME 18

Therapeutic interventions for Carcinoid Syndrome 22

Managing Carcinoid Syndrome through Dietary and Exercise Interventions 26

CHAPTER III: TACTICS TO CONQUER CARCINOID SYNDROME 33

Awareness of Carcinoid Syndrome 40

Assistance and guidance for individuals coping with Carcinoid Syndrome. 43

CHAPTER IV: CARCINOID SYNDROME: EXPECTED OUTCOME 46

Research and Future Advancements 49

Challenges Linked to Carcinoid Syndrome 53

CHAPTER V: NUTRITIOUS DISHES FOR CARCINOID SYNDROME 59

NUTRITIOUS BREAKFAST DISHES 59

Banana Bread Bundt Cake 59

Key Lime Waffles 63

4-Minute Mug Cinnamon Rolls 65

Lighter Pumpkin Bread 69

Microwaved Egg Breakfast Sandwich 71

Confetti Crullers 73

Whole Wheat Waffle Sticks 78

Breakfast Veggie Pocket.. 81

Strawberry Breakfast Muffins................................... 83

The Ultimate Waffle 86

Zucchini Cheddar Muffins 89

Berry-Stuffed French Toast For Two....................... 93

Banana Pancakes.. 96

Sheet Tray Pancakes 99

Healthier Frozen Breakfast Burritos 101

Lemon Blueberry Coffee Cake................................ 105

Rainbow Croissants... 111

Loaded Savory Vegetable Crostata........................ 117

Egg-In-A-Hole Sweet Potato Nests........................ 124

Hacked Croissant Donuts.. 127

NUTRITIOUS DISHES FOR LUNCH 130

Chicken Pot Pie Soup 130

Chickpea Garlic "Meat"balls.......................... 133

Birria Tacos 136

Meal-Prep Garlic Chicken And Veggie Pasta...... 144

Classic Meatloaf 148

The Creamiest Butter Chicken 151

Instant Pot Mac & Cheese............................ 161

Deep Dish Pizza With Sausage And Mushrooms

.... 163

Black Bean & Tofu "Meat"balls 170

Arugula, Peach, And Goat Cheese Flatbread...... 172

Salted Honey Apple Brie Grilled Cheese 177

Korean Corn Dogs.. 179

Shrimp Kale Caesar Salad 186

60-Minute Lasagna 191

Steak And Cheddar Grilled Cheese Sandwiches 196

Tandoori Turkey 200

Oxtail Beignets 212

Malaysian Chicken Curry Laksa (Laksa Lemak) 221

Torta Ahogada 228

Peanut Butter & Jelly Spiders................................ 236

Meal Prep Pesto Chicken Pasta 238

NUTRITIOUS DISHES FOR EVENING MEALS 240

One-Pot Pesto Chicken Pasta................................ 241

Crunchy Avocado Tuna Wraps........................... 244

One-Pan Chicken Adobo................................... 247

The Best Homemade Pizza.............................. 249

Pesto Garden Pasta For The Whole Family 256

Pumpkin Sage Pasta 259

Country Fried Steak And Gravy........................... 261

Baked Chicken Parmesan 265

Tuna Burgers 268

BBQ Chicken Pita Pizza 271

Easy Slow Cooker Mozzarella-Stuffed Meatballs And Sauce 273

Pulled Pork-Stuffed Milk Buns 277

Healthy Veggie Curry With Garlic Naan 281

Copycat Campfire Chicken 288

Honey Mustard Glazed Ham 292

Homemade Chicken Shawarma 295

Lasagna-Stuffed Peppers 300

Chicken Curry Naan Bowls................................... 304

Garlic Herb-Crusted Roast Rack Of Lamb 313

Beet Gnocchi 316

NUTRITIOUS DISHES FOR APPETIZERS 321

Rainbow Veggie Pinwheels................................... 321

Chicken And Spinach Pull-Apart Bread 324

Zucchini Carrot Fritters 328

The Ultimate Dinner Rolls.................................... 331

Onion Rings.. 335

White Pizza Dip 338

Loaded Sweet Potato Skins 341

Brazilian Chicken Croquettes (Coxinha).............. 344

Chicken Alfredo Bread Boat.................................. 348

Curry Puffs 2 Ways.. 353

Pakistani-Style Veggie Pakoras.............................. 357

Pizza Popovers.. 361

Queso Lava Cakes 364

Gravy-Stuffed Cheddar Biscuit Bombs 369

Chili Mac 'N' Cheese Pops................................... 375

Shamrock Empanadas.. 382

Nashville Hot Fried Pickles................................. 389

Pretzels And Beer Cheese Spread 399

Baked Delicata Squash Rings With Honey Mustard

Dipping Sauce 403

Blossoming Onion Lotus 407

SECTION 6: FINALLY! 412

To the Reader, From the Author 414

INTRODUCTION

Carcinoid Syndrome, a rare condition, manifests due to neuroendocrine tumors (NETs) that overproduce hormones, notably serotonin. These tumors can arise throughout the body, though they are commonly found in the digestive system, lungs, and pancreas. The symptoms associated with Carcinoid Syndrome are diverse, including flushing, diarrhea, wheezing, stomach discomfort, and fatigue.

Diagnosing Carcinoid Syndrome typically involves a comprehensive approach, encompassing physical examinations, blood tests, and imaging scans. Treatment strategies are tailored to the specific characteristics of the tumor, such as its size, location, and the severity of symptoms. However, it is estimated that neuroendocrine tumors (NETs), which may lead to carcinoid syndrome, occur in approximately 6-7 occurrences per 100,000 individuals annually.

On a global scale, there appears to be an increasing incidence of NETs, possibly due to advancements in diagnostic techniques. The prognosis for patients with carcinoid syndrome varies depending on several factors, including the tumor's location and size, the presence of metastases, and the individual's overall health. Nevertheless, with appropriate therapy and care, many patients with carcinoid syndrome can maintain a high quality of life and engage in their daily activities without significant hindrance.

CHAPTER I: WHAT EXACTLY IS CARCINOID SYNDROME?

Carcinoid syndrome, a term previously associated with carcinoid tumors, is a multifaceted collection of symptoms that may signal the presence of neuroendocrine tumors (NETs), which originate from specialized neuroendocrine cells within the body. These cells are dispersed throughout various organs and tissues, fulfilling crucial roles in regulating the production and release of hormones that coordinate a multitude of bodily activities. Hormones serve as the messengers of the body, orchestrating intricate processes and signaling pathways that dictate physiological responses.

The development of NETs arises from the aberrant proliferation and division of these neuroendocrine cells, leading to the formation of tumors. These tumors, when located in the gastrointestinal tract, can elicit carcinoid syndrome by releasing an array of substances, including serotonin and other chemical mediators, into the bloodstream. This biochemical cascade initiates a domino effect of physiological changes, giving rise to a diverse spectrum of symptoms that characterize carcinoid syndrome.

The manifestations of carcinoid syndrome encompass a broad range of clinical presentations, extending from facial flushing and diarrhea to cardiac complications such as heart valve damage and pulmonary issues like bronchoconstriction. Additionally, patients may experience fluctuations in blood pressure, abdominal pain, and even neurological symptoms due to the systemic effects of the released substances.

Understanding and effectively managing carcinoid syndrome require a comprehensive comprehension of its underlying mechanisms, encompassing the intricate interplay between neuroendocrine cells, hormone secretion, and bodily functions. Moreover, the diagnosis and treatment of carcinoid syndrome necessitate a multidisciplinary approach, involving collaboration between oncologists, endocrinologists, gastroenterologists, and other specialists to tailor interventions that address the diverse array of symptoms and mitigate the impact of NETs on overall health and quality of life.

Causes of Cardiovascular Syndrome

The onset of Circadian Syndrome can be attributed to the suppression of specific hormones and substances by carotid tumors. These tumors, known as low-growing neuroendocrine tumors or carcinoid tumors, originate from the nerve cells within the system. With the capacity to release various substances into circulation such as ergotamine, hydroxyzine, and phytoandrogens, these tumors pose a complex challenge to the body's hormonal equilibrium.

The exact etiology of carcinoid tumors remains elusive, although prevailing theories suggest a correlation with genetic mutations occurring within the cells of the neuroendocrine system. Furthermore, the development of carcinoid tumors has been associated with several risk factors, including a familial history of neuroendocrine cancers like carcinoid tumors, multiple endocrine disorders such as MEN1, and exposure to certain toxins or chemicals like pesticides, herbicides, or industrial compounds.

While many individuals with cardiac tumors may not manifest symptoms of Circadian Syndrome, in other instances, these tumors may secrete sufficient hormones and substances to induce symptoms such as diarrhea, abdominal pain, wheezing, and palpitations.

The underlying mechanisms of Circadian Syndrome are not fully elucidated; however, it is conjectured that tumors within the neuroendocrine system precipitate the sequestration of hormones. Older adults are more predisposed to such tumors, which can either be sporadic or inherited. Risk factors may heighten the likelihood of developing the disorder, such as exposure to certain chemicals or a family history of Circadian Syndrome.

When the digestive tract excessively produces and transmits hormones to the liver, it triggers carcinoid syndrome. Normally, the liver regulates this flow even when a neuroendocrine tumor enhances hormone synthesis. However, if the gastrointestinal tract generates an excess of hormones or if a neuroendocrine tumor in the liver impedes its processing and elimination, the system may become overwhelmed with hormones, precipitating a cardiac condition termed syndrome of undetermined origin.

A family history of neuroblastoma or other neuroendocrine tumors can increase the risk of developing carcinoid syndrome. Carcinoid tumors may occasionally have a hereditary component, whereby genetic alterations can be passed down through families and predispose individuals to these tumors.

MEN1, a genetic condition, can elevate the risk of developing neuroendocrine tumors, including carcinoid tumors. Individuals with MEN1 harbor a mutation in the MEN1 gene, which typically regulates cell growth and division in the neuroendocrine system. Several neuroendocrine tumors, including carcinoid tumors, may arise due to MEN1 gene mutations.

Other genetic changes, such as those in the succinate dehydrogenase (SDH) gene and the von Hippel-Lindau (VHL) gene, have also been implicated in the emergence of cardiac malignancies.

It is imperative to discuss with healthcare providers about one's risk and any recommended screening or monitoring, especially if there is a family history of carcinoid tumors or other neuroendocrine tumors. Genetic testing may be advised in some scenarios to identify any unintended mutations that might increase the risk of developing carcinoid tumors or other neuroendocrine tumors.

Certain medical conditions, such as numerous endocrine disorders, Type 1 Neoplasia (MEN1), might be correlated with Circadian Syndrome. Rare genetic condition MEN1 can heighten the risk of several cancers developing in endocrine glands such as the pituitary, parathyroid, and pancreas.

People with MEN1 have a mutation in the MEN1 gene, which typically aids in regulating the growth and division of cells in the endocrine system. Many malignancies, including neuroendocrine tumors like cardiac tumors, may occur as a result of MEN1 gene mutations. Some medical conditions linked to the development of carcinoid tumors and carcinoid syndrome include Zöllinger-Ellison syndrome, which causes excessive stomach acid production leading to the growth of carcinoid tumors in the digestive system. A genetic disorder called neurofibromatosis type 1 can increase the risk of developing nervous system cancers, particularly neuroendocrine tumors.

The Carney triad, an uncommon syndrome, results in the growth of multiple tumors, including paragangliomas, pulmonary chlamydia, and gastrointestinal stromal tumors (GISTs).

It is crucial to speak with healthcare practitioners about any screening or monitoring that may be advised if one has a medical condition that might raise the risk of developing carcinoid tumors or Circadian Syndrome. Early identification and treatment of carcinoid tumors can improve outcomes and lower the risk of complications like carcinoid syndrome.

Exposure to certain toxins or chemicals, such as industrial chemicals, insecticides, or herbicides, has been linked to the formation of carcinoid tumors and carcinoid syndrome. However, there is limited evidence linking environmental exposure to carcinoid tumors, and further study is required to fully comprehend the role of environmental variables in the emergence of this illness.

According to certain studies, exposure to pesticides and herbicides may be associated with a higher risk of developing cancerous tumors, particularly in the digestive system. Several studies have suggested a possible connection between industrial chemical exposure, such as that from polychlorinated biphenyls (PCBs), and the development of neuroendocrine tumors, including carcinoid tumors.

It is crucial to remember that the evidence linking environmental exposures to carcinoid tumors and Circadian Syndrome is not definitive, and many other factors may have contributed to the development of these conditions. For advice on how to decrease exposure to environmental toxins or chemicals, as well as any screening or monitoring that may be advised, speak with healthcare practitioners if there are any concerns.

Indications of Cardinod Syndrome

The manifestations of Carcinoid Syndrome exhibit a spectrum of variations contingent upon the tumor's site within the body and the specific hormones it produces. Among these, flushing emerges as a predominant symptom, often accompanied by sensations of coldness, redness, or an itching sensation across the visage, neck, or chest. Additionally, diarrhea presents as a common symptom, manifesting in either watery or fatty consistency, often coupled with cramping or abdominal discomfort.

Respiratory challenges, including wheezing, may arise due to pulmonary complications or constriction of the airways. Concurrently, weakness or fatigue may be experienced alongside rapid heartbeat or palpitations. Less frequently observed symptoms encompass unexplained weight loss, nausea, and vomiting.

The earliest and most prevalent indicators of Carcinoid Syndrome typically involve uncomfortable flushing of the head and neck, coupled with watery diarrhea. Unfortunately, many of the symptoms associated with Carcinoid Syndrome overlap with those of other ailments, leading to potential misdiagnosis. Conditions such as menopause, Crohn's disease, and even irritable bowel syndrome (IBS) have been mistakenly identified as Carcinoid Syndrome.

Seeking medical attention is paramount if experiencing any of the following symptoms:

- Abdominal cramps and frequent, explosive diarrhea.

- Foul-smelling fatty stools.

- Edema or swelling of the legs and feet, indicative of potential heart failure.

- Respiratory distress and wheezing.

- Loss of libido or development of erectile dysfunction.

- Jaundice, characterized by yellowing of the skin and eyes.

- Feelings of drowsiness or anxiety, which may signal low blood pressure.

- Sensation of heart palpitations.

CHAPTER II: DIAGNOSIS OF CARCINOID SYNDROME

The diagnosis of Carcinoid Syndrome involves a comprehensive approach encompassing various medical evaluations and diagnostic procedures tailored to uncover and understand the intricacies of this complex condition. A crucial component in this diagnostic journey is the amalgamation of physical examinations, blood analyses, and imaging studies, each playing a pivotal role in elucidating the manifestations and underlying pathology associated with Carcinoid Syndrome.

Physical examinations serve as the initial gateway for clinicians to observe and assess potential signs and symptoms indicative of Carcinoid Syndrome. During these assessments, healthcare providers meticulously scrutinize patients for telltale signs such as abdominal discomfort or tenderness, which may hint at the presence of carcinoid tumors. Moreover, observable phenomena like flushing or skin discoloration and respiratory irregularities such as wheezing or shortness of breath can offer valuable diagnostic clues, further guiding the diagnostic process. Additionally, the presence of edema or swelling in specific regions of the body may serve as a visible marker of the syndrome, aiding in its identification during physical examinations.

Complementing physical examinations, blood tests stand as a cornerstone in the diagnostic arsenal against Carcinoid Syndrome, furnishing clinicians with invaluable insights into the biochemical landscape of the patient's physiology. Through the analysis of blood samples, healthcare providers can discern the levels of various hormones and biomarkers that may be indicative of carcinoid tumors or associated syndromes. For instance, measurements of serotonin, chromogranin A, and 5-HIAA can provide critical information regarding tumor activity and hormone secretion patterns, facilitating the diagnostic process. Furthermore, comprehensive blood panels can offer insights into liver function and metabolic dynamics, crucial facets in understanding the systemic impact of Carcinoid Syndrome on overall health.

However, the diagnostic journey does not culminate with blood tests alone. Imaging studies play an indispensable role in providing clinicians with a visual roadmap of the internal landscape, aiding in the localization, characterization, and staging of carcinoid tumors. Techniques such as computed tomography

(CT) scans, magnetic resonance imaging (MRI), and positron emission tomography (PET) scans offer unparalleled insights into tumor morphology, distribution, and potential metastasis, guiding treatment decisions and prognostic evaluations. Additionally, specialized imaging modalities like octreotide scans and endoscopy provide clinicians with targeted approaches to visualize and characterize tumors, further enhancing diagnostic precision.

It is imperative to recognize that the diagnostic journey for Carcinoid Syndrome necessitates a multidimensional approach, wherein each facet of evaluation serves as a vital piece of the diagnostic puzzle. By integrating physical examinations, blood analyses, and imaging studies, clinicians can navigate the complexities of Carcinoid Syndrome with precision and efficacy, ultimately facilitating timely interventions and improved patient outcomes. Therefore, collaborative discussions between patients and healthcare providers regarding the selection and interpretation of diagnostic modalities are paramount, ensuring a comprehensive and patient-centered approach to diagnosis and management.

Therapeutic interventions for Carcinoid Syndrome

The treatment landscape for carcinoid syndrome is multifaceted and tailored to individual cases, with considerations spanning tumor size, location, symptom severity, and patient-specific factors. Among the arsenal of therapeutic approaches, surgery often emerges as a frontline option, particularly for localized tumors where excision may be curative or aimed at debulking to alleviate symptoms and impede disease progression.

In cases where surgical intervention is warranted, the precise modality varies depending on tumor characteristics and patient health status. Surgical strategies range from complete tumor resection, termed curative surgery, to debulking procedures aimed at maximal tumor removal while preserving organ function and quality of life. Advanced techniques such as laparoscopic surgery may be employed in select cases to minimize invasiveness and enhance postoperative recovery.

Complementary to surgical management, a spectrum of therapies exists to address carcinoid symptoms and disease progression. Chemotherapy, while less commonly utilized due to the relative insensitivity of carcinoid tumors, may be considered when tumors have metastasized beyond surgical reach. However, its systemic effects and potential side effects necessitate careful patient selection and monitoring.

Targeted therapy represents a burgeoning frontier in carcinoid syndrome management, leveraging medications designed to selectively target cancer cells while sparing healthy tissues. These agents may disrupt hormonal pathways crucial for tumor growth or directly inhibit molecules vital for cancer cell survival. For instance, somatostatin analogs mimic the action of naturally occurring somatostatin to modulate hormone production, thereby alleviating symptoms. Other targeted therapies, such as tyrosine kinase inhibitors and mTOR inhibitors, hold promise in halting disease progression by interfering with specific cellular signaling pathways.

Navigating the complexities of targeted therapy necessitates close collaboration between patients and specialized healthcare providers versed in neuroendocrine tumor management. Tailoring treatment regimens to individual tumor profiles and patient needs underscores the importance of a multidisciplinary approach in optimizing therapeutic outcomes and enhancing quality of life for those affected by carcinoid syndrome.

Managing Carcinoid Syndrome through Dietary and Exercise Interventions

Implementing alterations to both dietary habits and lifestyle choices holds significant potential in effectively managing the symptoms associated with carcinoid syndrome. These adjustments can encompass a multifaceted approach involving mindful eating practices, hydration strategies, exercise regimens, stress management techniques, and smoking cessation efforts. By adopting these changes, individuals grappling with carcinoid syndrome can potentially experience a noticeable improvement in their quality of life.

Dietary modifications constitute a cornerstone of symptom management in carcinoid syndrome.

Optimal dietary choices may include consuming smaller, more frequent meals to alleviate diarrhea episodes, steering clear of trigger foods such as alcohol, sugary items, and caffeinated beverages like coffee, while prioritizing the intake of fiber-rich foods like fruits, vegetables, and whole grains. Tracking food intake and its impact on symptoms empowers individuals to make informed dietary decisions, enhancing their ability to mitigate discomfort and manage the condition effectively.

Avoidance of specific trigger foods remains paramount in symptom management. Foods such as alcohol, coffee, spicy dishes, and high-fat items have been implicated in exacerbating symptoms characteristic of carcinoid syndrome. By maintaining awareness of personal dietary triggers and making conscientious choices to limit or eliminate their consumption, individuals can exert a degree of control over symptom severity and frequency.

Furthermore, adopting a pattern of consuming smaller, more frequent meals throughout the day can aid in preventing symptom exacerbation. By distributing food intake evenly across the day, the digestive system is less likely to become overwhelmed, reducing the likelihood of experiencing distressing symptoms such as stomach cramping and diarrhea. It's recommended to aim for approximately 5-6 small meals spaced out every 2-3 hours, thereby also promoting stable blood sugar levels.

When increasing fiber intake—a practice beneficial for regulating bowel movements and managing diarrhea—it's crucial to do so gradually and cautiously. Selecting soluble fiber sources, such as certain grains, beans, peas, and fruits like pears and apples, can aid in digestion while minimizing the risk of gastrointestinal discomfort. Additionally, maintaining adequate hydration is essential, as it can help prevent constipation, a potential side effect of a high-fiber diet.

Staying hydrated is paramount for individuals with carcinoid syndrome, particularly given the propensity for dehydration associated with diarrhea. Consuming an ample amount of fluids throughout the day, primarily through water consumption, is imperative. Additionally, alternatives like coconut water, known for its electrolyte content, can aid in replenishing lost fluids and minerals. Employing hydration-enhancing practices such as using a straw or incorporating hydrating foods into the diet further supports this endeavor.

Regular physical activity also plays a pivotal role in symptom management, as it contributes to overall health improvement and stress reduction. Engaging in exercise routines tailored to individual capabilities and preferences can yield substantial benefits, including symptom alleviation and enhanced well-being. Prior consultation with a healthcare provider is advisable before embarking on any new exercise regimen, especially for individuals with pre-existing health conditions.

Effectively managing stress is another vital component of mitigating symptoms associated with carcinoid syndrome. Utilizing relaxation techniques such as deep breathing, meditation, and yoga can help lower stress levels and foster a sense of calmness and well-being. Additionally, seeking social support and guidance from mental health professionals can aid in developing coping strategies tailored to individual needs, enhancing overall resilience and quality of life.

Lastly, quitting smoking is paramount for individuals with carcinoid syndrome, as smoking can exacerbate symptoms and complicate treatment outcomes. Despite the challenges associated with smoking cessation, numerous resources and support systems are available to assist individuals in this endeavor, including nicotine replacement therapies and counseling services. Quitting smoking not only improves overall health but also enhances the effectiveness of medications used to manage carcinoid syndrome.

CHAPTER III: TACTICS TO CONQUER CARCINOID SYNDROME

Implementing alterations to both dietary habits and lifestyle choices holds significant potential in effectively managing the symptoms associated with carcinoid syndrome. These adjustments can encompass a multifaceted approach involving mindful eating practices, hydration strategies, exercise regimens, stress management techniques, and smoking cessation efforts. By adopting these changes, individuals grappling with carcinoid syndrome can potentially experience a noticeable improvement in their quality of life.

Dietary modifications constitute a cornerstone of symptom management in carcinoid syndrome.

Optimal dietary choices may include consuming smaller, more frequent meals to alleviate diarrhea episodes, steering clear of trigger foods such as alcohol, sugary items, and caffeinated beverages like coffee, while prioritizing the intake of fiber-rich foods like fruits, vegetables, and whole grains. Tracking food intake and its impact on symptoms empowers individuals to make informed dietary decisions, enhancing their ability to mitigate discomfort and manage the condition effectively.

Avoidance of specific trigger foods remains paramount in symptom management. Foods such as alcohol, coffee, spicy dishes, and high-fat items have been implicated in exacerbating symptoms characteristic of carcinoid syndrome. By maintaining awareness of personal dietary triggers and making conscientious choices to limit or eliminate their consumption, individuals can exert a degree of control over symptom severity and frequency.

Furthermore, adopting a pattern of consuming smaller, more frequent meals throughout the day can aid in preventing symptom exacerbation. By distributing food intake evenly across the day, the digestive system is less likely to become overwhelmed, reducing the likelihood of experiencing distressing symptoms such as stomach cramping and diarrhea. It's recommended to aim for approximately 5-6 small meals spaced out every 2-3 hours, thereby also promoting stable blood sugar levels.

When increasing fiber intake—a practice beneficial for regulating bowel movements and managing diarrhea—it's crucial to do so gradually and cautiously. Selecting soluble fiber sources, such as certain grains, beans, peas, and fruits like pears and apples, can aid in digestion while minimizing the risk of gastrointestinal discomfort. Additionally, maintaining adequate hydration is essential, as it can help prevent constipation, a potential side effect of a high-fiber diet.

Staying hydrated is paramount for individuals with carcinoid syndrome, particularly given the propensity for dehydration associated with diarrhea. Consuming an ample amount of fluids throughout the day, primarily through water consumption, is imperative. Additionally, alternatives like coconut water, known for its electrolyte content, can aid in replenishing lost fluids and minerals. Employing hydration-enhancing practices such as using a straw or incorporating hydrating foods into the diet further supports this endeavor.

Regular physical activity also plays a pivotal role in symptom management, as it contributes to overall health improvement and stress reduction. Engaging in exercise routines tailored to individual capabilities and preferences can yield substantial benefits, including symptom alleviation and enhanced well-being. Prior consultation with a healthcare provider is advisable before embarking on any new exercise regimen, especially for individuals with pre-existing health conditions.

Effectively managing stress is another vital component of mitigating symptoms associated with carcinoid syndrome. Utilizing relaxation techniques such as deep breathing, meditation, and yoga can help lower stress levels and foster a sense of calmness and well-being. Additionally, seeking social support and guidance from mental health professionals can aid in developing coping strategies tailored to individual needs, enhancing overall resilience and quality of life.

Lastly, quitting smoking is paramount for individuals with carcinoid syndrome, as smoking can exacerbate symptoms and complicate treatment outcomes. Despite the challenges associated with smoking cessation, numerous resources and support systems are available to assist individuals in this endeavor, including nicotine replacement therapies and counseling services. Quitting smoking not only improves overall health but also enhances the effectiveness of medications used to manage carcinoid syndrome.

Implementing comprehensive dietary and lifestyle modifications tailored to individual needs and circumstances can significantly contribute to effectively managing the symptoms of carcinoid syndrome. By prioritizing mindful eating, hydration, exercise, stress management, and smoking cessation, individuals can take proactive steps towards enhancing their well-being and quality of life. Collaboration with healthcare providers specializing in the treatment of neuroendocrine tumors ensures personalized guidance and support throughout this journey.

Awareness of Carcinoid Syndrome

Advocacy plays a pivotal role in the ongoing battle against Carcinoid Syndrome and in the continual quest for advancements in research and enhanced treatment modalities. Numerous advocacy organizations, such as the Carcinoid Cancer Foundation and the Neuroendocrine Tumor Research Foundation, are dedicated to providing invaluable support to patients and their families grappling with this challenging illness. These organizations serve as pillars of information dissemination, advocacy, and emotional sustenance for those navigating the complexities of Carcinoid Syndrome.

Their efforts span a spectrum of activities aimed at bolstering research endeavors to refine treatments and improve patient outcomes, fostering greater awareness of the illness, and advocating for policy reforms to ensure access to comprehensive care for individuals affected by Carcinoid Syndrome. Among the multifaceted dimensions of advocacy, these groups engage in lobbying endeavors at local, national, and international levels, alongside offering vital informational resources.

The Carcinoid Cancer Foundation, the Neuroendocrine Tumor Research Foundation, and the Healing NET Foundation stand as just a few examples of the advocacy organizations committed to assisting those impacted by Carcinoid Syndrome and their support networks. Their missions extend beyond providing assistance; they actively champion policy changes while serving as informative hubs and resource repositories.

Individuals living with Carcinoid Syndrome also play an essential role in advocacy efforts, advocating for themselves and their communities by sharing their personal experiences, participating in research studies, and contributing to fundraising initiatives aimed at bolstering awareness and research endeavors. Advocacy endeavors further entail engaging with policymakers and healthcare professionals to enhance access to care, promote research initiatives, and foster a deeper understanding of the unique needs of individuals living with autoimmune diseases like lupus and scleroderma. Through collaborative advocacy efforts, strides can be made in alleviating the burdens of Carcinoid Syndrome and improving the quality of life for those affected by it.

Assistance and guidance for individuals coping with Carcinoid Syndrome.

Advocacy plays a pivotal role in the ongoing battle against Carcinoid Syndrome and in the continual quest for advancements in research and enhanced treatment modalities. Numerous advocacy organizations, such as the Carcinoid Cancer Foundation and the Neuroendocrine Tumor Research Foundation, are dedicated to providing invaluable support to patients and their families grappling with this challenging illness. These organizations serve as pillars of information dissemination, advocacy, and emotional sustenance for those navigating the complexities of Carcinoid Syndrome.

Their efforts span a spectrum of activities aimed at bolstering research endeavors to refine treatments and improve patient outcomes, fostering greater awareness of the illness, and advocating for policy reforms to ensure access to comprehensive care for individuals affected by Carcinoid Syndrome. Among the multifaceted dimensions of advocacy, these groups engage in lobbying endeavors at local, national, and international levels, alongside offering vital informational resources.

The Carcinoid Cancer Foundation, the Neuroendocrine Tumor Research Foundation, and the Healing NET Foundation stand as just a few examples of the advocacy organizations committed to assisting those impacted by Carcinoid Syndrome and their support networks. Their missions extend beyond providing assistance; they actively champion policy changes while serving as informative hubs and resource repositories.

Individuals living with Carcinoid Syndrome also play an essential role in advocacy efforts, advocating for themselves and their communities by sharing their personal experiences, participating in research studies, and contributing to fundraising initiatives aimed at bolstering awareness and research endeavors. Advocacy endeavors further entail engaging with policymakers and healthcare professionals to enhance access to care, promote research initiatives, and foster a deeper understanding of the unique needs of individuals living with autoimmune diseases like lupus and scleroderma. Through collaborative advocacy efforts, strides can be made in alleviating the burdens of Carcinoid Syndrome and improving the quality of life for those affected by it.

CHAPTER IV: CARCINOID SYNDROME: EXPECTED OUTCOME

The prognosis and outlook for individuals diagnosed with Carcinoid Syndrome hinge upon a multifaceted interplay of various factors, encompassing not only the specific location and size of the tumor but also the intensity of symptoms manifested and the overall health condition of the patient. This syndrome, a result of neuroendocrine tumors, presents a spectrum of outcomes ranging from manageable to potentially life-altering, contingent upon the responsiveness to treatment and the implementation of lifestyle modifications.

A pivotal aspect in the management of Carcinoid Syndrome lies in the diligent management of symptoms and the prevention of recurrence, both of which necessitate consistent monitoring and vigilant follow-up treatment. The trajectory of this syndrome's progression is intricately tied to the severity of the underlying tumor and the patient's individual response to therapeutic interventions. For those fortunate individuals who receive timely and appropriate medical care, the prognosis often holds promise, with a notable 65–75% five-year survival rate reported.

However, in instances where the tumor has metastasized to other regions of the body or when diagnosis occurs at later stages, the prognosis can be considerably graver. Moreover, the presence of certain malignancies or underlying medical disorders can heighten the likelihood of complications, further complicating the prognosis.

In navigating the complexities of Carcinoid Syndrome, collaboration between patients and their healthcare providers is paramount. By collectively crafting a comprehensive treatment plan and committing to regular follow-up care, individuals afflicted by this syndrome can effectively monitor symptoms and swiftly address any potential complications as they arise. With diligent care and proactive management, many individuals diagnosed with Carcinoid Syndrome can aspire to lead fulfilling, active lives, underscoring the importance of personalized, patient-centered approaches in optimizing outcomes and enhancing quality of life.

Research and Future Advancements

Research efforts dedicated to understanding the complexities surrounding Carcinoid Syndrome are in a perpetual state of motion, characterized by a multifaceted approach aimed at unraveling its intricate causes and advancing treatment modalities to enhance patient well-being. At the forefront of this endeavor lies an array of pioneering investigations geared towards the development of innovative pharmaceutical interventions with the overarching goal of improving clinical outcomes.

One significant avenue of exploration revolves around the refinement of diagnostic methodologies, as current techniques often fall short in providing precise and timely identification of the syndrome. Manifesting symptoms that lack distinct clarity and laboratory findings that may not always yield definitive conclusions underscore the pressing need for more sophisticated diagnostic tools capable of swiftly and accurately pinpointing the ailment.

Moreover, researchers are diligently delving into the realm of targeted therapies, recognizing the limitations of existing treatments which may prove ineffective for certain individuals. This pursuit entails the meticulous design of therapeutic agents specifically tailored to selectively target tumor cells while mitigating adverse effects, thereby heralding a new era of personalized medicine.

However, amidst these endeavors, the fundamental mechanisms underpinning the onset and progression of Carcinoid Syndrome remain shrouded in ambiguity, prompting investigators to embark on a quest to decipher the genetic and molecular intricacies orchestrating the development of carcinoid tumors. By unraveling these intricacies, researchers hope to unveil novel therapeutic targets that could revolutionize treatment paradigms.

Furthermore, the quest for prevention strategies occupies a pivotal position within the research landscape, as scientists strive to elucidate the various risk factors contributing to the onset of Carcinoid

Syndrome and devise proactive measures aimed at thwarting its emergence. The interplay between dietary habits, lifestyle choices, and environmental factors in fostering the growth of cancerous tumors constitutes a focal point of inquiry, offering potential avenues for preventive interventions.

Equally imperative is the pursuit of strategies geared towards ameliorating the debilitating symptoms associated with Carcinoid Syndrome, thereby enhancing the quality of life for affected individuals. Recognizing the profound impact that this syndrome exerts on patients' well-being, efforts are underway to address not only the physical manifestations but also the emotional and psychological ramifications of the disease. This entails the development of more efficacious approaches for managing symptoms such as diarrhea and flushing, alongside providing comprehensive support to address the holistic needs of patients navigating this challenging medical terrain.

Challenges Linked to Carcinoid Syndrome

Untreated Carcinoid Syndrome can lead to a cascade of serious health consequences, rippling through various bodily systems with potentially dire outcomes. One of the primary dangers lies in the impact on the cardiovascular system, particularly with regards to heart valve damage attributed to heightened levels of serotonin in the bloodstream. This biochemical imbalance can trigger a thickening and stiffening of the heart valves, impeding their flexibility and compromising efficient blood flow. In extreme cases, this can culminate in heart failure, a condition fraught with life-threatening implications.

Moreover, the repercussions of Carcinoid Syndrome extend beyond the cardiovascular realm, infiltrating other vital organs and bodily functions. Intestinal obstruction, liver damage, and uncontrollable bleeding stand as ominous possibilities, casting a shadow over the overall health landscape of those affected by this syndrome.

Among the complex interplays of Carcinoid Syndrome with bodily functions, diseases of the heart and lungs emerge as prominent concerns. The presence of cancerous endocrine tumors can induce not only heart valve damage but also respiratory issues, manifesting as wheezing and shortness of breath owing to the overproduction of hormones. Serotonin, in particular, emerges as a key player in exacerbating lung issues and potentially compromising cardiac integrity.

The intricate dance between serotonin and cardiovascular health further unravels as it instigates thickening and scarring of the heart valves, predominantly affecting the right-sided valves. This pathological process can usher in valvular stenosis or regurgitation, impairing the heart's efficacy in pumping blood, consequently precipitating symptoms such as fatigue, shortness of breath, and peripheral edema.

Furthermore, the surplus serotonin wreaks havoc on the pulmonary vasculature, constricting blood arteries within the lungs and precipitating pulmonary hypertension. This condition, characterized by abnormally elevated blood pressure within the lung vasculature, manifests through symptoms like dyspnea, chest discomfort, and profound fatigue, imposing significant burdens on the afflicted individuals.

In light of these grave health threats, individuals grappling with Carcinoid Syndrome necessitate vigilant monitoring of their cardiac and pulmonary statuses to promptly detect and address any burgeoning complications. Treatment modalities encompass a spectrum ranging from symptomatic management with medications to surgical interventions like valve replacement to mitigate the progression of heart failure.

Beyond the cardiovascular and pulmonary ramifications, the gastrointestinal manifestations of Carcinoid Syndrome loom large, predominantly in the form of debilitating diarrhea. This persistent symptom not only predisposes individuals to dehydration but also precipitates electrolyte imbalances and nutritional deficiencies if left unchecked. Mitigating strategies involve meticulous fluid management, dietary modifications, and judicious medication use under the guidance of healthcare professionals.

Concurrently, the specter of abdominal discomfort and agony looms large, often stemming from the cramping and distress associated with diarrhea bouts. Identifying trigger foods and implementing dietary adjustments emerge as pivotal strategies in assuaging gastrointestinal distress, supplemented by pharmacological interventions aimed at alleviating pain and discomfort.

Malabsorption emerges as another formidable challenge, underpinning the vicious cycle of malnutrition and weight loss in individuals grappling with Carcinoid Syndrome. The compromised absorptive capacity of the intestines precipitates a slew of symptoms ranging from diarrhea to abdominal pain, underscoring the imperative of tailored dietary regimens and, in severe cases, intravenous nutritional support to redress the nutritional deficits.

Carcinoid Syndrome precipitates a multifaceted assault on various physiological systems, necessitating a comprehensive and multidisciplinary approach encompassing meticulous monitoring, targeted interventions, and holistic supportive care to mitigate its deleterious effects and optimize the quality of life for affected individuals.

CHAPTER V: NUTRITIOUS DISHES FOR CARCINOID SYNDROME

NUTRITIOUS BREAKFAST DISHES

Banana Bread Bundt Cake

What You Need -

for 10 servings

CAKE

nonstick cooking spray, for greasing

5 ripe bananas

3 large eggs

¾ cup nonfat greek yogurt(215 g)

½ cup honey(170 g)

1 ½ teaspoons vanilla extract

2 ¼ cups whole wheat flour(290 g)

1 ½ teaspoons baking soda

1 cup walnuts(100 g), roughly chopped, plus more for topping

FROSTING

2 cups powdered sugar(240 g)

2 tablespoons plain nonfat greek yogurt

Method

Preheat the oven to 350°F (180°C). Grease a bundt pan with nonstick spray.

In a large bowl, mash the bananas. Add the eggs, yogurt, honey, and vanilla and whisk to combine.

Add the flour and baking soda and stir with a rubber spatula to incorporate. Fold in the walnuts.

Pour the batter into the prepared bundt pan. Smooth the top with a spatula.

Bake for about 50 minutes, or until a toothpick inserted in the center comes out clean. Baking times may vary, so keep an eye on the bread.

Invert the cake onto a wire rack set over a baking sheet and let cool completely.

Make the frosting: In a small bowl, mix together the powdered sugar and 2 tablespoons of Greek yogurt. Add more yogurt as needed until your desired consistency is reached.

Pour the frosting over the bread. Quickly sprinkle more walnuts on top before the frosting sets.

Slice and serve.

Enjoy!

Key Lime Waffles

What You Need -

for 6 servings

WAFFLES

2 eggs

1 ⅓ cups whole milk(320 mL)

1 container Oikos Greek Yogurt Key Lime, (5.3-ounce)

1 tablespoon sugar(15 g)

1 tablespoon baking powder(12 g)

½ teaspoon kosher salt(2.5 g)

2 cups flour(250 g)

TOPPING

1 container Oikos Greek Yogurt Key Lime, (5.3-ounce)

2 teaspoons lime zest(2 g)

1 tablespoon maple syrup(21 g)

Lime slice, for garnish

Method

In a bowl, whisk together eggs, whole milk, and Oikos Greek Yogurt Key Lime. Add in sugar, baking powder, kosher salt, and flour. Whisk until all the dry ingredients are incorporated.

Coat waffle iron with nonstick spray. Heat up iron. Pour a heaping ½ cup of batter in the center of the iron. Close and cook for 3–4 minutes, or until golden brown and cooked through. Repeat with the rest of the batter.

In a small bowl, whisk together Oikos Greek Yogurt Key Lime, lime zest, and maple syrup. Top waffles with a dollop and garnish with a lime slice.

Serve and enjoy!

4-Minute Mug Cinnamon Rolls

What You Need -

for 2 servings

FILLING

1 tablespoon unsalted butter

2 tablespoons brown sugar

½ teaspoon cinnamon

DOUGH

1 large egg

1 teaspoon vanilla extract

1 tablespoon granulated sugar

2 tablespoons whole milk

1 ½ cups pancake mix(180 g)

all purpose flour, for dusting

nonstick cooking spray, for greasing

2 teaspoons water

ICING

6 tablespoons powdered sugar

1 tablespoon whole milk

Method

Make the filling: In a small bowl, combine the melted butter, brown sugar, and cinnamon. Make the dough: In a medium bowl, whisk together the egg, vanilla, sugar, and milk until combined. Add the pancake mix and stir with a rubber spatula until mostly incorporated.

Turn the dough out onto a lightly floured surface and knead briefly until mostly smooth. Roll the dough out to an 8 x 6-inch rectangle.

Spread the filling over the dough. Starting with a long edge, tightly roll the dough into a log. Cut in half crosswise.

Grease 2 12-ounce mugs with nonstick spray. Place 1 cinnamon roll in each mug with the cut side facing up. Spoon 1 teaspoon of water into each mug. Working 1 at a time, microwave the cinnamon rolls on medium power for 1 minute and 45 seconds. Let cool for 1 minute.

Make the icing: In a small bowl, stir together the powdered sugar and milk until smooth.

Drizzle the icing over the cinnamon rolls before serving.

Enjoy!

Lighter Pumpkin Bread

What You Need -

for 12 servings

2 eggs

½ cup oil(120 mL)

1 cup pumpkin puree(225 g)

⅔ cup honey(226 g)

2 tablespoons water

1 ¾ cups whole wheat flour(225 g)

1 ½ teaspoons ground cinnamon

1 ½ teaspoons ground nutmeg

½ teaspoon ground ginger

1 teaspoon baking soda

1 pinch salt

Method

Preheat the oven to 350°F (180°C).

In a large bowl, combine the eggs, oil, pumpkin, honey, and water, and whisk until thoroughly combined.

Sprinkle the whole wheat flour, cinnamon, nutmeg, ginger, baking soda, and salt over the wet What You Need - and fold until the batter is well combined.

Pour the batter into a greased loaf pan and smooth the top into an even layer.

Bake for 1 hour, or until a toothpick inserted into the center comes out clean.

Let the loaf cool in the pan for 10 minutes before carefully unmolding.

Let the loaf sit at room temperature for at least 1 hour before slicing.

Enjoy!

Microwaved Egg Breakfast Sandwich

What You Need -

for 1 serving

1 egg

salt, to taste

pepper, to taste

1 whole wheat english muffin

tomato, to serve

fresh spinach, to serve

avocado, to serve

Method

Crack the egg into the mug then season with salt and pepper.

Beat the egg.

Place the mug in the microwave and cover with a wet paper towel.

Cook for approximately 30-40 seconds.

Toast the English muffin. Then top with the egg, tomato, avocado, and spinach.

Enjoy!

Confetti Crullers

What You Need -

for 16 crullers

1 cup unsalted butter(230 g), 2 sticks, cubed

1 ¼ cups water(300 mL)

1 ¼ cups milk(300 mL)

¼ cup granulated sugar(50 g)

1 teaspoon salt

1 cup all-purpose flour(125 g)

½ cup whole wheat flour(65 g)

2 teaspoons baking powder

5 large eggs

2 teaspoons vanilla extract, divided

⅓ cup rainbow sprinkles(65 g), plus more for topping

8 cups canola oil(1.9 L)

GLAZE

4 cups powdered sugar(480 g), sifted

4 tablespoons milk

1 teaspoon vanilla extract

3 tablespoons cream cheese, softened

SPECIAL EQUIPMENT

large star piping tip

deep fry thermometer

Method

In a large pot over medium heat, combine the butter, water, milk, sugar, and salt. Whisk until the butter is melted and the mixture is steaming, about 5 minutes.

Quickly whisk the all-purpose and whole wheat flours and the baking powder into the hot milk mixture. Continue cooking, stirring constantly, for 5 more minutes. Remove the pot from heat and stir with a spatula to cool the dough.

When the dough is no longer hot to the touch, add the eggs one at a time, stirring to incorporate before adding the next.

Add the vanilla and sprinkles and stir to distribute evenly.

Transfer the dough to a piping bag or zip-top bag fitted with a large star tip.

On a parchment-lined baking sheet, pipe 4-inch (10-cm) circles of dough. Chill in the freezer until solid, about 20 minutes.

Meanwhile, make the glaze: In a large bowl, combine the powdered sugar, milk, vanilla, and cream cheese. Whisk until smooth and runny. Set aside.

Heat the oil in a large pot until it reaches 350°F (180°C).

Carefully add the crullers to the hot oil. Fry about 3 at a time for 4-5 minutes, flipping halfway, until golden brown. The fried crullers should feel much lighter than they were originally. Transfer the fried crullers to a wire rack set over a baking sheet.

While still warm, dip one side of the crullers in the glaze. Return to the wire rack and allow excess glaze to drip off. Top with sprinkles.

Enjoy!

Whole Wheat Waffle Sticks

What You Need -

for 8 servings

2 large eggs

1 cup whole greek yogurt(245 g)

½ cup milk(120 mL), of choice

¼ cup oil(60 mL)

2 tablespoons maple syrup, plus more for dipping

1 ⅓ cups whole wheat flour(165 g)

1 ½ teaspoons baking powder

½ teaspoon baking soda

powdered sugar, for dusting

Method

Preheat the Griddler, fitted with the waffle plates, to 375°F (190°C), and grease with nonstick spray.

Whisk the eggs in a large mixing bowl until smooth.

Add the Greek yogurt and whisk again until smooth.

Whisk in the milk, oil, and maple syrup.

Add the flour, baking powder, and baking soda, and whisk together until the batter is smooth and well combined.

Use a 1-cup (130 G) measuring cup to pour batter onto the Griddler.

Cook for 10 minutes, until the waffle has puffed up and is golden brown. Transfer the waffle to a cutting board and repeat with the remaining batter.

Cut the waffles into sticks.

Sprinkle with powdered sugar and serve with maple syrup.

Enjoy!

Breakfast Veggie Pocket

What You Need -

for 1 serving

2 teaspoons olive oil

½ red bell pepper, sliced

¼ cup canned black bean(40 g), drained and rinsed

¼ cup frozen corn(45 g), thawed

½ small yellow onion, thinly sliced

2 eggs

¼ teaspoon salt

¼ teaspoon ground black pepper

¼ cup shredded cheddar cheese(25 g)

1 whole wheat tortilla, medium

Method

Heat olive oil in a nonstick skillet over medium heat.

Add the bell pepper, black beans, corn, and onions, and cook until caramelized, about 5 minutes.

Remove the vegetables from the pan and set aside.

Reduce heat to low, and eggs, and sprinkle with salt and pepper. Cook, stirring constantly, until barely set, about 2 minutes.

Place the vegetables, scrambled eggs, and cheese in the center of a tortilla, and fold the sides into the center, completely covering the filling.

Add the quesadilla, seam side down, to the skillet and cook over medium heat until the outside is toasted and cheese is melted.

Enjoy!

Strawberry Breakfast Muffins

What You Need -

for 6 servings

1 cup whole wheat flour(115 g)

1 ¼ teaspoons baking powder

¼ teaspoon salt

1 cup strawberry(175 g), diced

2 eggs, room temperature

⅓ cup honey(115 g)

½ cup greek yogurt(140 g), room temperature

3 tablespoons coconut oil, melted, plus more for greasing

Method

Preheat oven to 375°F (190°C).

In a large mixing bowl, whisk together the eggs, yogurt, honey, strawberries, and coconut oil until well combined.

Add the flour, baking powder, and salt, and fold the batter together using a rubber spatula. Stop folding once all of the dry ingredients have disappeared into the batter.

Using a medium ice cream scoop, pour one scoop full of batter into each well of a greased muffin tin.

Bake for for 20-25 minutes, until a toothpick inserted in the center of a muffin comes out clean.

Enjoy!

The Ultimate Waffle

What You Need -

for 4 servings

2 cups all purpose flour(250 g)

2 teaspoons baking powder

1 teaspoon kosher salt

1 cup whole milk(240 mL)

½ cup buttermilk(120 mL)

4 tablespoons unsalted butter, melted and
cooled

½ teaspoon vanilla extract

2 large eggs, separated

⅓ cup sugar(65 g)

nonstick cooking spray, for greasing

butter, for serving

maple syrup, for serving

Method

Preheat a waffle iron to medium-high.

In a large bowl, whisk together the flour, baking powder, and salt. Make a well in the center and pour in the milk, buttermilk, melted butter, vanilla, and egg yolks. Whisk until the batter just comes together (there will be some lumps).

Add the egg whites to a medium bowl and beat with an electric hand mixer until foamy. With the mixer running, gradually add the sugar and continue beating until stiff peaks form. Gently fold the egg whites into the batter until just combined.

Spray the heated waffle iron with nonstick cooking spray. Ladle the batter into the waffle iron, close the lid, and cook according to manufacturer's instructions until the waffle is golden brown and crisp, 5–6 minutes. Transfer the waffle to a plate and repeat with the remaining batter.

Serve the waffles hot, with butter and maple syrup alongside.

Enjoy!

Zucchini Cheddar Muffins

What You Need -

for 12 muffins

nonstick cooking spray, for greasing

2 cups whole wheat flour(260 g)

1 teaspoon baking powder

½ teaspoon baking soda

1 teaspoon kosher salt

1 teaspoon black pepper

1 pinch sugar

3 large eggs

1 cup buttermilk(240 mL), 1 cup (240 ml) milk mixed with 1 teaspoon white vinegar

5 tablespoons unsalted butter, or olive oil

1 cup zucchini(150 g), shredded

1 cup carrot(110 g), shredded

1 cup shredded cheddar cheese(100 g), plus more for topping

¼ cup chives(10 g), thinly sliced

Method

Preheat the oven to 350°F (180°C). Grease a 12-cup muffin tin with nonstick spray.

Make the batter: In a large bowl, stir together the whole wheat flour, baking powder, baking soda, salt, pepper, and sugar. Set aside.

In a medium bowl, whisk together the eggs, buttermilk, and butter.

Add the zucchini, carrot, cheddar cheese, and chives the egg mixture and stir to combine.

Pour the egg mixture into the dry ingredients and fold to combine, being careful not to overmix.

Using an ice cream scoop, divide the batter between the muffin cups, filling almost completely.

Sprinkle more cheddar cheese on top of the muffins.

Bake for 18 minutes, rotating the muffin tin halfway through baking, until browned on top and a toothpick inserted in the center of a muffin comes out clean.

Let cool for 10 minutes before removing the muffins from the tin. Serve or store in the refrigerator for up to 5 days.

Enjoy!

Nutrition, per muffin - Calories: 182, Total fat: 10 grams, Sodium: 433 mg, Total carbs: 17 grams, Dietary fiber: 3 grams, Sugars: 2 grams, Protein: 7 grams

Berry-Stuffed French Toast For Two

What You Need -

for 2 servings

FILLING

1 cup raspberry(125 g)

1 cup blackberry(125 g)

2 tablespoons maple syrup, divided

1 tablespoon black raspberry liqueur

4 oz cream cheese(115 g), softened

FRENCH TOAST

4 slices brioche bread

½ cup whole milk(120 mL)

1 large egg, beaten

2 tablespoons black raspberry liqueur

½ teaspoon salt

2 tablespoons butter

WHIPPED CREAM

½ cup heavy cream(120 mL)

1 tablespoon maple syrup

Method

Make the filling: Add the raspberries, blackberries, black raspberry liqueur, and 1 tablespoon of maple syrup to a large bowl. Stir and let sit for 10 minutes for the berries to macerate.

In a medium bowl, mix together the cream cheese and remaining tablespoon of maple syrup until smooth.

Spread the filling evenly over the 4 slices of bread. Arrange some of the berries on 2 slices of the bread and top with the other slices of bread. Press to seal the pieces together.

In a shallow dish, whisk together the milk, egg, black raspberry liqueur, and salt.

Melt the butter on a griddle or in a large skillet over medium heat. Quickly dip both sides of the bread pockets in the milk mixture, then transfer to the pan and fry on each side for about 3 minutes, until golden brown.

In a large bowl, beat the heavy cream until soft peaks form. Add the maple syrup and continue beating until the cream holds medium peaks.

Serve the stuffed French toast with a dollop of maple whipped cream and a scoop of macerated berries with their soaking liquid.

Enjoy!

Banana Pancakes

What You Need -

for 6 pancakes

1 banana, mashed, extra to garnish

½ cup applesauce(130 g)

2 cups almond milk(480 mL)

1 teaspoon vanilla extract

1 cup whole wheat flour(130 g)

3 teaspoons baking powder

1 pinch salt

EGG SUBSTITUTE OPTIONS (CHOOSE ONE)

1 tablespoon chia seed

1 tablespoon ground flaxseed, mixed with 3 tablespoons of water

½ banana, mashed

Method

Mash one banana to substitute for egg.

For chia or ground flax seeds, mix with water and let rest for 5-10 minutes.

Add to the other wet What You Need -. Mix well.

Add flour, baking powder, and salt to wet ingredients until well combined.

Measure out ¼ cup (60 ml) of batter and add to a skillet over low heat.

When bubbles start to form and edges start to come off the pan, flip the pancake.

Cook an additional 2-3 minutes. Repeat with remaining batter.

Enjoy!

Sheet Tray Pancakes

What You Need -

for 8 servings

1 ½ cups whole wheat flour(195 g)

1 teaspoon baking powder

⅔ cup almond milk(160 mL)

1 ¼ cups unsweetened applesauce(280 g)

2 eggs

1 teaspoon vanilla extract

blueberry, to taste

strawberry, to taste

dark chocolate chip, to taste

banana, to taste

Method

Preheat oven to 425°F (220°C).

In a bowl, mix whole wheat flour and baking powder.

Add in milk, applesauce, egg, and vanilla extract. Mix until well combined.

Pour pancake mix on a greased baking sheet and evenly spread out.

Add desired toppings onto the whole pan or place in different corners for a variety.

Bake for 15 minutes.

Cut into squares. Serve now or freeze for up to a month.

Enjoy!

Healthier Frozen Breakfast Burritos

What You Need -

for 6 servings

4 slices turkey bacon

1 sweet potato, peeled and diced

1 red bell pepper, diced

6 cups fresh spinach(240 g), sauteed

6 eggs, beaten

olive oil, or oil of choice

salt, to taste

pepper, to taste

shredded cheese, of choice, to taste

whole wheat tortilla

Method

In a large skillet over medium heat, cook turkey bacon according to package instructions. Remove and set to the side.

Using the same skillet, add diced sweet potatoes and season with salt and pepper. Cook until soft. Remove from pan and set aside.

Add diced red bell peppers and cook until softened. Remove from pan and set aside.

Cook spinach, then set aside.

Reduce heat to medium-low and pour in beaten eggs. Remove from pan once cooked.

To assemble the burritos, place down parchment paper, then put the tortilla on top.

Add scrambled eggs, sweet potatoes, spinach, bell pepper, turkey bacon, and cheese.

Fold the left and right side of the burrito in, then fold the bottom up and roll tightly.

Roll burrito into parchment paper.

Serve now or place into a bag or reusable container.

Transfer to the freezer. Freeze for up to 1 month.

To reheat, remove burrito from parchment paper and wrap in a damp paper towel.

Microwave for 3 minutes or until warm.

Rest for one minute.

Enjoy!

Lemon Blueberry Coffee Cake

What You Need -

for 6 servings

nonstick cooking spray, for greasing

STREUSEL TOPPING

¼ cup granulated sugar(50 g)

¼ cup light brown sugar(50 g)

¼ cup all purpose flour(30 g)

¼ cup unsalted butter(55 g), cut into small pieces, room temperature

LEMON- BLUEBERRY COFFEE CAKE

1 cup fresh blueberry(100 g)

1 ½ cups all purpose flour(185 g), divided, plus 1 tablespoon

1 ½ teaspoons baking powder

½ teaspoon kosher salt

½ cup unsalted butter(115 g), room temperature

¾ cup granulated sugar(150 g)

2 large eggs, room temperature

1 teaspoon vanilla extract

3 tablespoons fresh lemon juice

1 tablespoon lemon zest

½ cup whole milk(120 mL), room temperature

LEMON GLAZE

1 ½ cups powdered sugar(165 g)

1 teaspoon lemon zest

2 tablespoons lemon juice

1 tablespoon whole milk, plus more as needed

Method

Preheat the oven to 350°F (180°C). Grease an 8½ x 4½-inch (20 cm x 11 cm) loaf pan with nonstick spray. Line the pan with a piece of parchment paper so there's overhang on both of the long sides.

Make the streusel topping: In a medium bowl, combine the granulated and brown sugars, flour, and butter. Mix together with a fork or with your fingers until crumbly and the butter is broken down into pea-sized pieces, being careful not to overmix. Set aside.

Make the coffee cake: Add the blueberries to a medium bowl and toss with 1 tablespoon of flour. This will prevent the blueberries from sinking to the bottom of the pan while baking. Set aside.

In a large bowl, whisk together the remaining 1½ cups (155 G) flour, the baking powder, and salt.

In a separate large bowl, cream the butter and granulated sugar with an electric hand mixer on medium speed until pale and fluffy, about

4 minutes. Add the eggs, 1 at a time, making sure the first egg is fully incorporated before adding the next. Mix in the vanilla, lemon juice and zest, and milk until fully combined.

Add the dry ingredients to the wet What You Need - and mix on low speed until fully combined. Add the blueberries to the batter and carefully fold with a rubber spatula to incorporate.

Pour the batter into the prepared loaf pan and spread evenly. Sprinkle the streusel topping evenly over the top.

Bake the coffee cake for 45–50 minutes, or until a toothpick inserted into the center comes out clean.

While the cake bakes, make the lemon glaze: In a medium bowl, whisk together the powdered sugar, lemon zest, lemon juice, and 1 tablespoon of milk until the sugar is dissolved. Add more milk, 1 tablespoon at a time, until the glaze reaches your desired consistency.

Let the cake cool in the pan for 10–15 minutes, then use the parchment sling to remove the cake from the pan. Drizzle the cake with the glaze before slicing with a serrated knife and serving.

Enjoy!

Rainbow Croissants

What You Need -

for 10 servings

⅔ cup whole milk(170 mL)

⅔ cup water(170 mL)

5 cups unbleached all-purpose flour(600 g), plus more for dusting

¼ cup granulated sugar(45 g)

1 tablespoon kosher salt

1 tablespoon instant dry yeast

3 tablespoons unsalted european-style butter, cubed, softened

5 food colorings, different colors

1 ¼ cups unsalted european-style butter(275 g), shaped into an 8X6-in (20x15-cm) rectangle, cold

1 large egg, beaten

SPECIAL EQUIPMENT

food-safe glove

Method

In a large bowl, combine the milk and water.

On top of the liquid, add the flour, sugar, salt, yeast, and cubed butter.

Mix just until the dough comes together, but don't overmix.

Set aside ¼ of the dough and transfer the rest to a lightly floured surface. Knead until the flour is fully incorporated. Shape into a ball, place in a large bowl, cover with plastic wrap, and let rest at room temperature for 2 hours.

Divide the reserved quarter of dough into 5 equal pieces. Add a few drop of different colored food coloring to each one.

Wearing food-safe gloves so you don't stain your skin, work each color into the dough.

Shape the colored dough into balls, place on a plate, and cover with plastic. Let rest for 2 hours at room temperature.

Transfer the large piece of rested dough to a parchment-lined baking sheet. Shape into an

8x11-inch (20x27 cm) rectangle, cover with plastic wrap, and chill in the refrigerator overnight.

Transfer the colored dough to another parchment-lined baking sheet. Shape into 2x3-inch (5x7 cm) rectangles, cover with plastic wrap, and chill overnight.

Transfer the plain rested dough to a clean, lightly floured surface. Roll into a 16x8-inch (40x20 cm) rectangle. Pat the edges with a knife to straighten.

Place the butter rectangle at the center of the dough rectangle. Fold the top and bottom of the dough over to cover the butter, pinching the center seam and sides to seal.

Rotate 90° and roll out to a large rectangle, about 8x18 inches (20x45 cm). Flatten the edges.

Fold the top and bottom edges to meet in the center of the dough. Fold over once more, then freeze for 30 minutes.

Roll out the dough again to a large rectangle, about 24x8 inches (60x20 cm). Brush off any excess flour. Fold the dough in thirds, brush again, then freeze for another 30 minutes.

Cut the chilled, colored doughs in half lengthwise. Roll into ropes about 10 inches (25 cm) long.

Brush the ropes with water and line up together, in rainbow order or as desired. Press together. Lightly dust with flour and roll out into a rectangle roughly the same size as the plain dough.

Brush the plain dough with water, then lay on the colored dough sheet on top.

Roll out into a large, 13x21-inch (33x53 cm) rectangle and about ¼-inch (6 mm) thick.

Cut the dough into 10 triangles with bases that are about 4 inches (10 cm) wide.

Lay the dough triangles colored side down, and starting with the wide end, gently roll up.

Place the croissants on a parchment-lined baking sheet, seam-side down. Cover with plastic wrap and let proof at room temperature for 2 hours.

Preheat the oven to 400°F (200°C).

Brush the croissants with egg wash.

Bake for 20-25 minutes, until golden brown. Let cool on a wire rack.

Enjoy!

Loaded Savory Vegetable Crostata

What You Need -

for 8 servings

CRUST

¾ cup all purpose flour(95 g), plus more for dusting

¾ cup whole wheat flour(95 g)

½ teaspoon kosher salt

6 tablespoons unsalted butter, cubed and chilled

3 tablespoons cold water

FILLING

3 tablespoons olive oil, divided

6 cloves garlic, peeled and stems removed

1 large yellow onion, thinly sliced

1 ½ teaspoons kosher salt, divided

2 medium red potatoes, thinly sliced

⅓ cup water(80 mL)

¼ teaspoon red pepper flakes

2 rainbow swiss chards, stem and leaves separated, thinly sliced

8 oz goat cheese(225 g), room temperature

1 large egg, beaten

Method

Make the crust: In a large bowl, mix together the all-purpose flour, whole wheat flour, and salt. Add the butter and, using a pastry cutter, work it into the flour until only pea-sized pieces remain. Add the water, starting with 3 tablespoons, and mix the dough with your fingers until it is moist enough to hold together. Add more water as needed, 1 tablespoon at a time. Turn the dough onto a clean surface, form into a disc, and wrap with plastic wrap. Refrigerate for 30-60 minutes.

Preheat the oven to 375°F (190°C). Line a baking sheet with parchment paper.

While the dough is resting, make the filling: Add 2 tablespoons of olive oil and the garlic cloves to a large, high-walled skillet over medium heat. Cook for 3 minutes, until the garlic just begins to brown. Add the onion and ½ teaspoon of salt. Cook for 20-25 minutes, until the onion is caramelized. Remove from the pan and set aside to cool in a bowl. To the same pan, add the potatoes, ½ teaspoon of salt, and the water. Increase the heat to medium-high, cover, and cook for 3-5 minutes, until the potatoes are almost fully cooked and the water is nearly evaporated. Remove the lid and cook for 2 minutes more to completely evaporate the water. Remove potatoes from the pan and set aside to cool.

To the same pan, add the remaining tablespoon of olive oil, the red pepper flakes, and chard stems. Reduce the heat to medium and cook for 3 minutes, until the stems are softened. Add the chard leaves and remaining ½ teaspoon of salt and cook for 5 minutes, until wilted and reduced in volume by half. Remove the pan from the heat.

Remove the garlic cloves from the caramelized onions and transfer to a small bowl. Mash with the back of a fork, then add to the softened goat cheese and stir to combine.

Stir the onions into the pan with the sautéed chard.

Assemble the crostata: Roll the dough out on a lightly floured surface into a 12-inch (30 cm) wide circle, about ⅛ inch (3 mm) thick. Transfer the dough to the prepared baking sheet.

Spread ½ cup (110 G) of the garlic goat cheese over the center of the dough, leaving a 2-inch (50 cm) border around the edges. Arrange half of the potatoes, slightly overlapping, over the goat cheese, then top with half of the Swiss chard and onion mixture. Repeat with remaining potatoes and chard mixture.

Fold the edges of the crust up and over the filling to create a rustic look. Brush the crust with the beaten egg. Top with dollops of the remaining goat cheese.

Bake the crostata for 45-50 minutes, until the crust is golden brown.

Let cool for 10 minutes before slicing and serving.

Enjoy!

Egg-In-A-Hole Sweet Potato Nests

What You Need -

for 6 servings

1 large sweet potato

1 medium yellow onion

1 ½ teaspoons salt

1 teaspoon pepper

1 teaspoon garlic powder

3 tablespoons flour

7 eggs

3 tablespoons olive oil

bacon, crumbs, to taste

raspberry, to taste

banana, sliced, to taste, to garnish

spring onion, to taste, to garnish

Method

Peel the skin off the sweet potato, and coarsely grate on a box grater.

Peel the onion, and coarsely grate on a box grater.

Transfer the grated sweet potato and onion to a towel-lined bowl.

Gently twist the towel, squeezing the liquid into an empty bowl and discard.

Transfer the sweet potato and onion to a bowl, and sprinkle with salt, pepper, garlic powder, flour, and 1 egg. Gently stir to combine.

Form large flat patties with your hands, approximately ⅓ cup of mixture each.

Heat a 9 ½ -inch (24 cm) fry pan on medium heat and coat with oil.

Add the sweet potato patties. Fry for 2-3 minutes, then gently flip.

Immediately use a small cookie cutter to remove a hole in the middle of each fritter.

Crack an egg in the hole, add a pinch of salt and pepper, then cover.

Fry for 3-7 minutes, or until cooked to your preference.

Uncover and serve with desired garnishes.

Enjoy!

Hacked Croissant Donuts

What You Need -

for 12 donuts

DOUGH

all purpose flour, for dusting

2 packages frozen puff pastry, thawed

1 large egg, beaten

ICING

1 cup vanilla frosting(175 g)

1 tablespoon whole milk

Method

Line a baking sheet with parchment paper.

Lay a puff pastry sheet flat on a lightly floured surface. Use a pastry brush to cover the sheet completely with the beaten egg. Fold the sheet into thirds along the creases, like a letter, and place on the prepared baking sheet. Repeat with the remaining 3 sheets of puff pastry. Refrigerate until stiff and completely chilled, about 1 hour.

Preheat the air fryer to 350°F (180°C) for 20 minutes. Set a wire rack over a baking sheet.

Remove the puff pastry from the refrigerator and use a 3-inch round cutter to cut out 12 rounds, 3 per sheet. Use a 1-inch round cutter to cut out the center of each pastry round. Remove and discard the scraps, or air fry for chef's snacks.

Working in batches, place the donuts in the air fryer, spacing 1 inch apart, and cook until the donuts have puffed completely and are golden brown all over, about 15 minutes. Transfer to the wire rack.

Make the icing: In a medium bowl, stir together the frosting and milk until smooth. Transfer the mixture to a small piping bag and cut a hole in the tip. Pipe the icing on the top of the donuts.

Enjoy!

NUTRITIOUS DISHES FOR LUNCH

Chicken Pot Pie Soup

What You Need -

for 6 servings

1 onion, diced

4 stalks celery, diced

6 carrots, diced

1 clove garlic

3 tablespoons butter

¼ cup flour(30 g)

2 cups chicken stock(470 mL)

2 cups half & half(470 mL)

1 teaspoon pepper

1 teaspoon dried thyme

1 pinch ground nutmeg

1 cup frozen corn(175 g)

1 cup frozen peas(150 g)

1 whole rotisserie chicken

Method

Heat oil in large pot on medium high heat.

Bring in onion, celery, carrots, and garlic and cook until onions are translucent, about 5 minutes.

Stir in butter and melt.

Add in flour and stir until flour butter mixture coats vegetables and browns lightly.

Add the chicken stock and half and half and stir to combine.

Season with pepper, thyme, and nutmeg and allow to come to a boil.

Reduce the heat to medium-low and add in corn, peas, and chicken and fully incorporate.

Season with salt.

Optional - garnish with cookie sized pieces of pie crust.

Enjoy!

Chickpea Garlic "Meat"balls

What You Need -

for 4 servings

water, or cooking oil

1 small onion, diced

4 cloves garlic, minced

15.5 oz chickpeas(440 g), 1 can, rinsed and drained

½ cup whole wheat breadcrumbs(60 g)

2 teaspoons fresh parsley, chopped

1 teaspoon dried oregano

½ teaspoon salt

½ teaspoon pepper

½ teaspoon red pepper flakes, optional

1 egg

Method

Preheat oven to 375°F (190°C).

In a skillet over medium heat, add cooking oil or water and onions. Cook until onions are translucent, stirring occasionally.

Add the garlic and stir until fragrant. Transfer to a blender or food processor.

To the food processor, add the chickpeas, breadcrumbs, parsley, oregano, salt, pepper, red pepper flakes, and egg. Pulse until a dough forms.

Use your hands to form 1-inch (2-cm) balls from the chickpea mixture. Place in rows on a parchment paper-lined baking sheet.

Bake for 20 minutes, or until golden, flipping halfway.

Enjoy!

Birria Tacos

What You Need -

for 3 servings

BIRRIA

¼ cup kosher salt(25 g), plus 1 tablespoon

2 lb beef chuck roast(910 g), cut into 1 in (2.54 cm) pieces

1 lb bone in beef short ribs(425 g)

5 dried ancho chiles

5 dried guajillo chiles

2 dried morita chiles

warm water, for soaking

1 whole cinnamon stick

1 tablespoon whole coriander seeds

1 tablespoon whole black peppercorn

4 whole allspice berries

2 whole cloves

6 dried bay leaves

1 teaspoon mexican oregano

¼ cup canola oil(60 mL), plus 1 tablespoon, plus more as needed

1 large yellow onion, chopped

4 roma tomatoes, quartered

8 cloves garlic, roughly chopped

¼ cup apple cider vinegar(60 mL)

8 cups water(2 L)

1 package frozen banana leaves, thawed

TACOS

12 corn tortillas

1 lb shredded queso oaxaca(450 g)

red onion, pickled

Radish, sliced

fresh cilantro, chopped

Lime wedge

Method

Make the birria: Line a baking sheet with parchment paper

Arrange the chuck roast and short ribs on the prepared baking sheet. Sprinkle ¼ cup salt all over the beef, making sure to coat each piece completely. Refrigerate for at least 4 hours and up to overnight.

Add the ancho, guajillo and morita chiles to a medium heatproof bowl. Cover with warm water and soak until starting to soften, about 5 minutes. Remove the seeds and stems and set chiles aside.

In a medium skillet over medium heat, toast the cinnamon stick, coriander, black pepper, allspice, and cloves until fragrant, about 2 minutes. Transfer the toasted spices, bay leaves, and oregano to a spice grinder or high-powered blender and grind into a fine powder.

Preheat the oven to 300°F (150°C).

Remove the seasoned meat from the refrigerator and use paper towels to pat dry.

In a large Dutch oven or heavy-bottomed pot with a tight fitting lid, heat ¼ cup canola oil over medium-high heat. When the oil is shimmering, sear the seasoned meat on all sides until golden brown, working in batches if needed to avoid overcrowding the pot, about

20 minutes. Remove the meat from the pot and set aside. If the oil looks dark and burnt, discard and add ¼ cup fresh canola oil to the pot and return to medium-high heat.

Add the yellow onion, tomatoes, and remaining tablespoon of salt to the hot oil and cook until the onion begins to sweat, 5–7 minutes. Add the garlic and cook until fragrant, about 3 minutes.

Add the ground spices and continue cooking until aromatic, about 2 minutes.

Add the apple cider vinegar, water, seared meat, and chiles. Bring to a boil, then reduce the heat to medium-low and cover. Simmer until the stew begins to thicken and the chiles are completely softened, about 30 minutes.

Remove the chiles from the stew and transfer to a high-powered blender with about 2 cups of the broth. Blend until smooth, then pour back into the pot and stir to combine. Cover the stew with the banana leaves, then place the lid on top. Transfer the stew to the oven and continue cooking until the meat easily pulls away from the short ribs bones, about 90 minutes. If the meat has some resistance, cover and cook longer, until very tender.

Remove the stew from the oven and discard the banana leaves, then remove the meat from the pot and transfer to a large bowl. Use a pair of tongs and a fork to shred the meat to your desired texture. Reserve the broth (consomé).

Make the tacos: Heat the remaining tablespoon of canola oil in a large cast iron skillet over medium heat until shimmering. Dip a tortilla in the warm consomé, then lay flat in the hot oil. Add 2 tablespoons of queso Oaxaca to one half of the tortilla and about ¼ cup of the shredded beef to the other half. Fold the quesadilla shut and cook until the cheese begins to melt, about 1 minute. Flip the quesadilla and continue cooking until the tortilla is golden brown and crispy and the cheese is oozing from the edges, about 1 minute. Repeat with the remaining tortillas, cheese and birria.

Serve the tacos with the consomé alongside for dipping as well as pickled onions, sliced radishes, chopped fresh cilantro, and lime wedges.

Enjoy!

Meal-Prep Garlic Chicken And Veggie Pasta

What You Need -

for 4 servings

4 tablespoons olive oil, divided

1 lb chicken breast(455 g), diced

2 carrots, sliced

1 zucchini, sliced

1 yellow squash, sliced

4 cups fresh kale(270 g), chopped

2 cloves garlic, minced

3 cups whole grain whole wheat rotini pasta(600 g), cooked al dente according to package instructions

2 teaspoons dried oregano, divided

2 teaspoons salt, divided

2 teaspoons pepper, divided

Method

Heat a large skillet with 2 tablespoons of olive oil on medium-high heat.

Add in diced chicken breast, followed by 1 teaspoon salt, 1 teaspoon pepper, and 1 teaspoon oregano. Cook until no longer pink. Remove chicken from skillet and set aside.

Add carrots to skillet and sauté for 2-3 minutes until tender.

Add in zucchini and yellow squash, and sauté for an additional minute until they become slightly translucent.

Add in the kale, followed by 2 tablespoons olive oil, 1 teaspoon salt, and 1 teaspoon pepper. Sauté until kale begins to wilt.

Move veggies aside with spatula and add in garlic. Sauté for about 30 seconds and then combine with the veggies. (This works best if you add garlic to the center of the skillet where there is more heat.)

Add in the cooked rotini pasta and chicken, followed by 1 teaspoon oregano and mix until evenly incorporated. Remove skillet from heat.

If using plastic tupperware for your weekday meal prep, allow pasta to cool for about 10 minutes before filling the containers. Refrigerate up to 4 days.

Or serve immediately for a family dinner.

Enjoy!

Classic Meatloaf

What You Need -

for 6 servings

1 tablespoon olive oil, plus more for greasing

1 large yellow onion, diced

3 cloves garlic, minced

2 tablespoons tomato paste

1 cup panko bread crumbs(115 g)

1 cup whole milk(240 mL)

2 lb ground beef(910 g)

2 large eggs, beaten

½ cup roughly chopped fresh parsley(10 g)

1 tablespoon worcestershire sauce

½ teaspoon dried thyme

1 tablespoon kosher salt

1 teaspoon freshly ground black pepper

½ cup ketchup(120 mL)

Method

Preheat the oven to 350°F (180°C). Line a rimmed baking sheet with foil.

Heat the olive oil in a large pan over medium-high heat. Once the oil begins to shimmer, add the onion and cook, stirring often, until softened and golden brown, about 7 minutes. Add the garlic and cook, stirring constantly, until aromatic, about 1 minute. Add the tomato paste and cook, stirring often, until the tomato paste turns deep red in color, about 2 minutes. Remove the pan from the heat and let the onion mixture cool to room temperature.

In a large bowl, stir together the panko and milk. Add the ground beef, eggs, parsley, Worcestershire sauce, thyme, salt, pepper, and the onion mixture and use your hands to combine. Do not overmix!

Shape the beef mixture into a 10 x 5-inch loaf on the prepared baking sheet. Brush the top and sides with ketchup.

Bake the meatloaf until the top is browned and the internal temperature reaches 160°F (70°C), about 50 minutes.

Slice and serve.

Enjoy!

The Creamiest Butter Chicken

What You Need -

for 4 servings

GARAM MASALA

1 dried bay leaf

2 whole cinnamon sticks

1 teaspoon whole cloves

20 whole black cardamom pods

1 tablespoon whole black peppercorns

2 tablespoons whole cumin seeds

4 tablespoons whole coriander seeds

½ whole nutmeg pod

GINGER-GARLIC PASTE

1 2-inch piece of fresh ginger, peeled

6 cloves garlic

1 tablespoon olive oil

1 pinch kosher salt

MARINADE

1 teaspoon ground turmeric

1 ½ teaspoons ground cumin

1 ½ teaspoons ground coriander

1 teaspoon kosher salt

½ lemon, juiced

1 teaspoon Kashmiri red chile powder

½ cup full-fat greek yogurt(120 mL)

8 boneless, skinless chicken thighs, (about 2 pounds), cut into strips or cubes

GRAVY

4 tablespoons unsalted butter, divided

2 tablespoons olive oil

½ teaspoon whole cumin seeds

1 whole black cardamom pod

1 dried bay leaf

4 whole cloves

2 green chiles, finely chopped (optional)

½ teaspoon ground turmeric

1 large yellow onion, chopped

1 ½ teaspoons ground cumin

1 teaspoon Kashmiri red chile powder

1 ½ teaspoons ground coriander

2 ½ cups canned crushed tomatoes(500 g)

½ cup cashews(60 g)

kosher salt, to taste

½ cup water(120 mL)

2 tablespoons sugar

2 tablespoons heavy cream

1 tablespoon dried fenugreek leaves

1 tablespoon freshly ground cilantro

FOR SERVING (OPTIONAL)

cooked basmati rice

onion kulcha

garlic naan

roti

Paratha

SPECIAL EQUIPMENT

12-inch wooden skewer

Method

Make the garam masala: Add the bay leaf, cinnamon stick, cloves, cardamom pods, blcak peppercorns, cumin seeds, coriander seeds, and nutmeg to a medium skillet. Toast over medium heat for 1–2 minutes, until fragrant, but not burnt. Transfer the toasted spices to a plate and let cool.

Transfer the spices to an electric spice grinder or mortar and pestle and grind into a fine powder. The garam masala will keep in an airtight container in a cool, dark place for several months.

Make the ginger-garlic paste: Add the ginger, garlic, oil, and salt to a small food processor or blender and process into a smooth paste, scraping down the sides of the processor as needed.

Marinate the chicken: In a large bowl, whisk together the 2 tablespoons ginger-garlic paste, 2 teaspoons garam masala, the turmeric, ground cumin, ground coriander, salt, lemon juice, Kashmiri red chile powder, and Greek yogurt until well combined. Add the chicken and toss to coat, then cover the bowl with plastic wrap and refrigerate for at least 3 hours, but ideally overnight.

Add the wooden skewers to a large baking dish. Cover with enough water to completely submerge, then soak for at least 1 hour.

When ready to cook the chicken, arrange an oven rack in the highest position. Turn the oven to broil on high. Set a wire rack over a rimmed baking sheet.

Thread the chicken onto wooden skewers and set on the wire rack, spacing evenly. Broil for 15 minutes, until evenly browned and cooked through, turning the skewers every 5 minutes to ensure even cooking. Let cool slightly before removing chicken from the skewers. Set aside.

While the chicken cooks, make the gravy: In a large, high-walled skillet, melt together the butter and olive oil over medium heat. Add the cumin seeds, cardamom pod, bay leaf, cloves, green chiles, and turmeric and sauté for 1 minute, until fragrant. Add the onion and cook for about 5 minutes, until lightly browned. Add 2 tablespoons ginger-garlic paste and cook for another minute, until fragrant. Add the ground cumin, Kashmiri red chile powder, ground coriander, and 1½ teaspoons of garam masala and stir for 1 minute, until well combined.

Add the crushed tomatoes, cashews, and a pinch of salt and cook, stirring often, for 10–15 minutes, until the tomatoes are a deeper, dark red color and the cashews are soft.

Transfer the tomato mixture to a high-powered blender. Add ½ cup water and blend until completely smooth, adding up to ½ cup more water if needed. If your blender is not high-powered, strain the gravy through a fine-mesh sieve after blending for a smoother texture.

Wipe the pan clean, then return the gravy to the pan. Add the remaining 3 tablespoons of butter, the sugar, and the cooked chicken. Cover and cook over low heat for 10 minutes, until the chicken is warmed through. Stir in the heavy cream and fenugreek and season with more salt to taste.

Garnish the butter chicken with cilantro and serve with your choice of basmati rice, onion kulcha, naan, roti, or paratha.

Enjoy!

Instant Pot Mac & Cheese

What You Need -

for 4 servings

1 lb dried elbow macaroni(425 g)

4 cups water(960 mL)

2 teaspoons kosher salt

3 tablespoons unsalted butter

4 cups shredded cheddar cheese

¼ cup whole milk(60 mL)

fresh parsley, for garnish - optional - chopped

Method

Add the macaroni, water, and salt to the Instant Pot and stir to combine. Close the lid and set to pressure cook on high for 4 minutes. Once the timer goes off, set the Instant Pot to quick release.

Remove the lid, add the butter, and stir until melted. Add the cheddar cheese, then the milk, 1 tablespoon at a time, and stir until melted and creamy.

Garnish with parsley, if desired, and serve.

Enjoy!

Deep Dish Pizza With Sausage And Mushrooms

What You Need -

for 6 servings

DOUGH

1 ¼ cups warm water(300 mL)

2 teaspoons sugar

2 ¼ teaspoons active dry yeast

3 ¼ cups all purpose flour(405 g), plus more for dusting

¾ cup cornmeal(110 g)

2 teaspoons kosher salt

¼ cup unsalted butter(55 g), melted and cooled

olive oil, for greasing

SAUCE

2 cans whole San Marzano tomatoes

2 teaspoons sugar

¼ teaspoon red pepper flakes

2 teaspoons kosher salt

2 tablespoons olive oil

4 cloves garlic, grated

¼ cup fresh basil(10 g), sliced

ASSEMBLY

1 tablespoon unsalted butter

8 oz white mushroom(225 g), sliced

kosher salt, to taste

¼ teaspoon whole fennel seeds

4 oz Italian sausage(115 g)

16 oz shredded low moisture mozzarella cheese(455 g)

¼ cup shredded parmesan cheese(25 g)

Method

Make the dough: Add the warm water and sugar to a large liquid measuring cup. Sprinkle in the yeast and let bloom for 5 minutes, until foamy.

In a large bowl, whisk together the flour, cornmeal, and salt. Add the yeast mixture and melted butter, and stir with a rubber spatula until a shaggy dough forms.

Turn the dough out onto a floured surface and knead for about 5 minutes, until the dough comes together into a soft ball and bounces back when pressed with a finger. Grease a large bowl with olive oil. Then transfer the dough to the bowl, cover with plastic wrap, and let rise in a warm spot until doubled in size, 1–2 hours.

Make the sauce: Pour the tomatoes into a fine-mesh sieve set over a bowl. Let the juices drain. Then use your hands to gently crush tomatoes and let any excess liquid drip into a bowl. Discard the juices. Transfer the crushed tomatoes to a medium saucepan and add the sugar, red pepper flakes, salt, olive oil, and garlic. Stir to combine. Bring to low boil over medium heat and cook for 15 minutes, until most of the liquid has evaporated. Remove the pot from the heat and stir in the basil. Set aside to cool while you prepare the rest of the toppings.

Melt the butter in a medium skillet over medium-high heat. Add the mushrooms and cook, stirring occasionally, until browned, about 5 minutes. Season with salt and remove the pan from the heat.

Add the fennel seeds to a small dry skillet over medium heat. Toast until fragrant and starting to brown, 3–4 minutes. Transfer the fennel seeds to a cutting board and coarsely chop.

Add the fennel seeds to a medium bowl with the Italian sausage and mix to incorporate. Transfer the sausage to a large sheet of parchment paper. Top with another sheet of parchment and roll the sausage into a 9-inch patty.

Preheat the oven to 425°F (220°C).

. Once the dough has risen, turn out onto a lightly floured surface. Cut the dough in half. Wrap one half in plastic wrap, place in a resealable zip-top bag, and freeze for up to 1 month.

Generously grease a 10-inch cast iron skillet with olive oil all over the sides and bottom. Transfer the remaining dough to the pan and use your hands to press evenly against the bottom and up the sides.

Tear the mozzarella into pieces and evenly scatter over the dough. Top with the sautéed mushrooms, then the tomato sauce. Use the parchment to place the sausage patty on top of the sauce. Sprinkle with the Parmesan.

Place the skillet on a baking sheet to catch any drips. Then transfer to the oven and bake for 35–40 minutes, until the crust is lightly browned and the sausage is cooked through.

Let cool slightly. Then carefully remove the pizza from the skillet, slice, and serve.

Enjoy!

Black Bean & Tofu "Meat"balls

What You Need -

for 4 servings

1 package firm tofu, patted dry

15.5 oz black beans(440 g), 1 can, drained and rinsed

1 red onion, diced

1 cup spinach(40 g)

3 cloves garlic, minced

1 tablespoon tomato paste

1 dried oregano

½ teaspoon salt

½ teaspoon pepper

1 teaspoon paprika

2 cups whole wheat breadcrumbs(230 g)

1 egg

Method

Preheat oven to 375°F (190°C).

In a blender or food processor, add tofu, black beans, onion, spinach, garlic, and tomato paste, and blend until smooth. Transfer to a large bowl.

To the bowl, add the oregano, salt, pepper, paprika, breadcrumbs, and egg. Mix well until a dough forms.

Use your hands to form 1-inch (2-cm) balls from the black bean and tofu mixture. Place in rows on a parchment paper-lined baking sheet.

Bake for 20 minutes, or until golden, flipping halfway.

Enjoy!

Arugula, Peach, And Goat Cheese Flatbread

What You Need -

for 4 servings

DOUGH

¾ cup warm water(180 mL), plus 2 tablespoons

1 ½ teaspoons instant yeast

1 cup all purpose flour(125 g), plus more for dusting

1 cup whole wheat flour(130 g)

1 ½ teaspoons kosher salt

1 teaspoon olive oil, plus more for brushing

TOPPINGS

2 ½ tablespoons olive oil, divided

1 medium yellow onion, thinly sliced

¾ teaspoon kosher salt, divided

½ teaspoon black pepper

1 teaspoon balsamic vinegar

6 cups fresh arugula(120 g)

2 medium peaches, thinly sliced

4 oz goat cheese(115 g), crumbled

2 tablespoons balsamic glaze

Method

Make the dough: In a large bowl, combine the warm water, yeast, all-purpose and whole wheat flours, and salt. Mix with a rubber spatula until well-combined and the dough comes together into a ball.

Lightly dust a clean surface with flour, then turn the dough out and knead for 1–2 minutes to smooth and encourage gluten development. Shape the dough into a ball.

Drizzle the olive oil in the bowl. Add the dough and turn to coat in the oil. Cover with a kitchen towel and let rise for 1 hour, or until doubled in size.

Caramelize the onions: Heat 2 tablespoons of olive oil in a large pan over medium heat. Add the onion, ½ teaspoon salt, and the pepper. Sauté for 5 minutes, until slightly softened. Add the balsamic vinegar, stir, and reduce the heat to low. Cook for about 25 minutes more, until the onions are tender and caramelized. Remove the pan from the heat and set aside to cool.

Punch down the dough, then divide into 4 pieces. On a lightly floured surface, roll out each piece to an 8-inch (20 cm) round, about ⅛ inch (3 mm) thick.

Heat a grill pan over medium-high heat. Brush each side of the dough lightly with olive oil. One at a time, grill each flatbread for about 4 minutes on each side, until grill marks appear and the dough is cooked through.

Add the arugula to a medium bowl, along with the caramelized onions, remaining ½ tablespoon olive oil, and remaining ¼ teaspoon salt. Toss well.

Top each flatbread with some of the arugula mixture, 6 peach slices, and 1 ounce of crumbled goat cheese. Drizzle with the balsamic glaze.

Enjoy!

Salted Honey Apple Brie Grilled Cheese

What You Need -

for 2 servings

4 slices fruit and nut bread, or rustic bread of choice

2 tablespoons unsalted butter, room temperature

2 tablespoons whole-grain Dijon mustard

1 granny smith apple, halved, cored, and sliced 1/8–1/4-inch-thick

2 teaspoons honey, plus more serving

flaky sea salt, for sprinkling

8 oz brie cheese(225 g), rind removed and sliced

Method

Heat a large griddle or skillet over medium-low heat.

Spread the butter on one side of each slice of bread. Flip the bread over and spread the mustard on 2 slices, then layer the apple slices on top of the mustard. Drizzle the honey over the apples, then sprinkle with a pinch of flaky salt. Arrange the Brie on the other slices of bread. Close the sandwiches.

Transfer the sandwiches to the pan and cook until golden brown on each side and the cheese has melted, 7–9 minutes per side.

Remove the sandwiches from the pan and cut in half. Top with another drizzle of honey and a sprinkle of flaky salt. Serve immediately.

Enjoy!

Korean Corn Dogs

What You Need -

for 12 servings

canola oil, for frying

POTATOES

kosher salt, for boiling

1 ½ lb russet potato(650 g), peeled and cut into 1/4 in (6mm)

2 tablespoons all purpose flour

BATTER

2 cups all purpose flour(250 g)

3 tablespoons granulated sugar

1 tablespoon baking powder

½ teaspoon kosher salt

1 cup whole milk(240 mL), plus 3 tablespoons

1 large egg, beaten

ASSEMBLY

6 all-beef hot dogs, halved crosswise

2 shredded low moisture mozzarella cheeses, 8 ounce (225 g) blocks

2 cups panko breadcrumbs(225 g)

2 cups korean rice puffs(100 g)

¼ cup granulated sugar(50 g), for sprinkling

KETCHUP

yellow mustard

SPECIAL EQUIPMENT

12 wooden skewers

Method

Fill a large stock pot fitted with a deep-fry thermometer with canola oil. Heat the oil over medium-high heat until the temperature reaches 350°F (180°C). Reduce the heat to medium to maintain the temperature. Set a wire rack over a baking sheet and place it nearby.

Prepare the potatoes: Bring a large pot of salted water to a boil. Add the potatoes and blanch for 2 minutes, then drain and transfer to a medium bowl. Let cool to room temperature, 15–20 minutes. Once cooled, sprinkle the flour over the potatoes and toss until well coated, shaking off and discarding any excess.

Make the batter: In a medium bowl, whisk together the flour, sugar, baking powder, and salt. In a 2-cup liquid measuring cup, whisk together 1 cup of milk and the egg until well combined. Pour the wet What You Need - into the dry ingredients and whisk until combined. The batter should be fairly thick; if it is too thick to whisk, add more milk, 1 tablespoon at a time. Transfer the batter to a pint glass or another tall, narrow container. Refrigerate until ready to use.

Thread each hot dog half onto the pointy end of a skewer, cut-side up, pushing down to about 2 inches below the tip. Thread the mozzarella rectangles onto the skewers above the hot dogs so they are flush with the cut ends of the hot dogs and the tips of the skewers.

Add the panko, floured potatoes, and rice puffs to individual plates or small trays.

Working one at a time, dip a cheese and hot dog skewer into the cup with the batter, coating completely. Gently shake off any excess batter.

For the original dogs: Roll a battered dog in the panko bread crumbs until well coated, using your fingers to pack on the bread crumbs as needed.

For the potato dogs: Roll a battered dog in the floured potatoes, using your hands to pack on the potatoes to ensure they stick. Immediately roll the potato-coated dog in the panko bread crumbs until completely coated.

For the crispy rice dogs: Roll a battered dog in rice puffs until completely coated, using your fingers to pack on the puffs as needed.

Place the coated dogs in the hot oil, 2–3 at a time, and fry for 2–3 minutes, until golden brown and crispy, using tongs to turn as needed. Transfer to the wire rack and sprinkle all over with sugar (use tongs when turning; the sticks will be very hot). Repeat with the remaining corn dogs to make 4 of each kind.

To serve, drizzle ketchup and mustard over the corn dogs.

Enjoy!

Shrimp Kale Caesar Salad

What You Need -

for 6 servings

CAESAR DRESSING

1 large free-range egg

2 teaspoons dijon mustard

3 fillets anchovies

2 cloves garlic

1 cup extra virgin olive oil(240 mL)

1 tablespoon fresh lemon juice, to taste

kosher salt, to taste

freshly ground black pepper, to taste

CROUTONS

6 oz whole grain wheat bread(170 g), 1 loaf, cut into bite-size cubes

olive oil, to taste

1 teaspoon italian seasoning

1 pinch kosher salt

SHRIMP

1 lb wild-caught shrimp(455 g), (about 21 or 25) peeled and deveined

2 tablespoons olive oil

2 cloves garlic, minced

1 lemon, zested

kosher salt, to taste

freshly ground black pepper, to taste

SALAD

12 cups kale(120 g), mixed, stemmed and sliced into ribbons

kosher salt, to taste

1 avocado, pitted and thinly sliced

¾ cup pomegranate seeds(130 g)

½ cup parmesan cheese(50 g), shaved

Method

Make the dressing: Add the egg, Dijon mustard, anchovy fillets, and garlic to a blender. Blend for about 1 minute, until smooth and creamy. With the blender running, slowly pour in the olive oil and blend until thick and emulsified. Season the dressing to taste with lemon juice, salt, and pepper, and quickly pulse to incorporate. Set aside. The dressing can be made ahead. Store in the fridge in an airtight container for up to 4 days.

Make the croutons: In a 3-quart (3 L) mixing bowl, combine the bread, olive oil, and Italian seasoning. Toss to coat the bread cubes.

Heat a medium pan over medium heat. Add the bread cubes, in batches if necessary to keep from overcrowding the pan. Toast, tossing occasionally, until crispy and golden brown, about 5 minutes. Remove from the pan and season with salt. Set aside. The croutons can be made ahead. Store in an airtight container in a cool, dry place for up to 4 days.

Make the shrimp: In a medium bowl, combine the shrimp, olive oil, garlic, lemon zest, salt, and pepper. Toss to coat the shrimp.

Heat a medium skillet over medium-high heat. Working in batches, cook the shrimp for 2 minutes on each side, until pink and opaque. Remove from the pan.

Thoroughly wash and dry the kale. Add to a large bowl and season with salt. Gently massage the kale to break down some of the fibrous texture. Toss with a bit of dressing to coat the leaves, then add more to taste.

Add the croutons, shrimp, avocado, pomegranate seeds, and Parmesan. Toss well.

Divide between bowls and serve immediately.

Enjoy!

60-Minute Lasagna

What You Need -

for 4 servings

2 tablespoons extra virgin olive oil

1 small yellow onion, small diced

3 sprigs fresh thyme, leaves picked

3 garlics, minced

4 oz mild italian sausage(120 g), casings removed

1 jar marinara sauce

1 ½ teaspoons kosher salt, plus more for boiling

8 lasagna noodles

3 cups whole milk ricotta cheese(735 g)

1 cup fresh baby spinach(40 g), chopped

1 ½ cups shredded mozzarella cheese(150 g), divided

¾ cup grated parmesan cheese(90 g), divided

2 tablespoons fresh basil, plus whole leaves, for garnish

1 tablespoon fresh parsley, minced

2 large egg yolks

½ teaspoon freshly ground black pepper

Method

Preheat the oven to 400°F (200°C).

Bring a large pot of salted water to a rolling boil.

Heat 1 tablespoon of olive oil in a large pan over medium heat. Add the onion and sauté until translucent, about 5 minutes. Add the thyme leaves and garlic and cook until fragrant, about 1 minute. Add the sausage and use a wooden spoon to break into very small pieces. Cook until no longer pink, 4–5 minutes. Add the marinara sauce and stir to combine. Simmer for about 5 minutes, until warmed through and the flavors combine. Remove the pan from the heat.

Season the boiling water generously with salt. Add the lasagna noodles and remaining tablespoon of olive oil and cook for 9–10 minutes, or about 2 minutes less than the package instructions, until al dente. Drain and rinse under cold water to prevent the noodles from sticking together. Lay the noodles on a baking sheet or cutting board.

In a large bowl, stir together the ricotta, spinach, ¾ cup mozzarella, ½ cup Parmesan, the basil, parsley, 1½ teaspoons salt, and ½ teaspoon black pepper.

Spoon about 1 cup of the tomato sauce into the bottom of a large casserole dish and spread evenly.

Lay a lasagna sheet on a clean surface. Spread about ½ cup of ricotta mixture over the noodle in an even layer, leaving a ½-inch edge on one end. Roll up tightly toward the empty end and place the roll-up in the casserole dish, seam-side down. Repeat with the remaining noodles and filling.

Spoon about 2 tablespoons of sauce over each roll-up. Sprinkle the remaining ¾ cup mozzarella and remaining ¼ cup Parmesan evenly over the top.

Bake the lasagna roll-ups for about 20 minutes, until the cheese is melted and bubbling.

Garnish with fresh basil leaves and serve.

Enjoy!

Steak And Cheddar Grilled Cheese Sandwiches

What You Need -

for 2 servings

1 cup white wine vinegar(240 mL)

1 tablespoon kosher salt, plus more to taste

1 tablespoon whole black peppercorn

2 teaspoons red pepper flakes

4 medium carrots, cut into ½-inch (1.24 cm) wide sticks

2 cloves garlic, peeled and smashed

1 large shallot, thinly sliced

1 ¼ cups water(300 mL)

1 tablespoon vegetable oil

8 oz flank steak(225 g)

freshly ground black pepper, to taste

2 tablespoons unsalted butter

4 slices sourdough bread

2 cups shredded sharp cheddar cheese(200 g)

Method

In a medium saucepan, combine the vinegar, 1 tablespoon salt, the peppercorns, red pepper flakes, carrots, garlic, shallot, and water. Bring to a boil over high heat and cook, stirring to dissolve the salt, for 1 minute. Remove from the heat and let cool to room temperature, about 20 minutes. (If not using immediately, transfer the carrots and their brine to an airtight container and refrigerate for up to 2 weeks.)

Meanwhile, heat the vegetable oil in a large cast-iron skillet over high heat.

Season the steak with salt and pepper. Transfer to the skillet and cook, flipping halfway, until golden brown on the outside and medium-rare inside, 6–8 minutes total. Transfer to a cutting board and let rest for 10 minutes, then thinly slice against the grain.

Return the skillet to medium heat and add the butter. Once melted, add 2 slices of sourdough bread. Top each slice with ½ cup shredded cheddar, and cook, undisturbed, until the bread is golden brown and toasted on the bottom and the cheese begins to melt, about 3 minutes. Divide the sliced steak between each slice of bread in the skillet, then top each with ½ cup of the remaining cheese and another slice of bread. Flip the sandwiches, cover the pan with a lid, and cook until the cheese has fully melted and the other side of the bread is golden brown and toasted, 2–3 minutes more.

Transfer the sandwiches to a cutting board and wrap each in foil. Serve with the pickled carrots alongside.

Enjoy!

Tandoori Turkey

What You Need -

for 12 servings

TANDOORI SPICE BLEND

4 cinnamon sticks, broekn into 1in (2.54 cm) pieces

¼ cup whole coriander(10 g)

3 tablespoons whole cumin seeds

3 whole mace blades

1 ½ tablespoons whole fenugreek seeds

1 tablespoon whole black cardamom pod

1 tablespoon whole green cardamom pods

1 tablespoon whole black peppercorn

1 tablespoon whole clove

3 tablespoons kashmiri chile powder

1 tablespoon ground ginger

1 tablespoon garlic powder

2 teaspoons freshly grated nutmeg

YOGURT MARINADE

32 oz plain full-fat greek yogurt(955 g)

¼ cup lemon juice(60 mL)

¼ cup kosher salt(30 g)

1 tablespoon grated fresh ginger

1 tablespoon grated garlic

TURKEY

1 turkey, thawed

TANDOORI GHEE

1 ½ cups ghee(325 g), clarified butter

2 teaspoons kosher salt

FOR ROASTING

2 lemons, quartered

1 head garlic, halved crosswise

4 fresh bay leaves

1 piece fresh ginger, sliced into 1/2 in thick rounds

½ bunch fresh cilantro

3 cups chicken stock(720 mL)

GRAVY

¼ cup all purpose flour(25 g), plus 2 tablespoons

3 cups reserved turkey drippings(720 mL), fat separated and discarded, warmed, or chicken stock

fresh cilantro, chopped

lime, quartered

Method

Make the tandoori spice blend: Set a medium skillet over medium-low heat and let the pan warm for a few minutes. Working one spice group at a time, toast the cinnamon sticks, coriander seeds, cumin seeds, mace blades (if using), fenugreek seeds, black and green cardamom pods, black peppercorns, and cloves in the warm skillet until each spice is fragrant and lightly browned, a few minutes per spice. Transfer the toasted spices to a plate or small tray while you toast the remaining spices. Let cool to room temperature.

Set a mesh strainer over a medium bowl. Once all of the whole spices have cooled, transfer to a high-powered blender or spice grinder (working in batches, if needed) and grind the spices into a fine powder. Pour the ground spices into the strainer and sift into the bowl below. Return any larger pieces to the blender and re-grind and sift into the bowl.

Add the Kashmiri chile powder, ground ginger, garlic powder, and nutmeg to the bowl with the ground spices and mix well to combine (if using ground mace, add here). Transfer the mixture to an airtight container and store in a cool, dry place until ready to use. The spice mixture will keep for up to 2 weeks.

Make the yogurt marinade: In a medium bowl, whisk together the yogurt, ¾ cup of the tandoori spice blend, the lemon juice, salt, ginger, and garlic until smooth.

Remove the innards from the turkey and discard (or save for another use). Pat the turkey dry all over with paper towels. Place the turkey in a bowl large enough to fit the bird, then pour the yogurt marinade all over the turkey. Use your fingers to gently loosen the turkey skin, starting from the top of the cavity and working your way toward the breasts and down toward the legs, being careful not to tear the skin. Use your hands to work the marinade underneath the skin and all over the entire bird. Once well-coated, cover the bowl with plastic wrap and refrigerate for at least 3 hours, preferably overnight.

While the turkey is marinating, make the tandoori ghee: Add the ghee to a small saucepan and cook over medium heat for 2–3 minutes, until hot. Add 2 tablespoons of the tandoori spice blend (it should sizzle lightly once it touches the ghee), then stir to incorporate and remove the pot from the heat. Stir in the salt. Transfer ¼ cup of the ghee to a small bowl and set aside to use for the gravy. Carefully pour the remaining 1¼ cups of ghee into a heat-proof container.

After marinating, remove the turkey from the refrigerator and let sit at room temperature for 2–3 hours before cooking.

Arrange a rack in the lower-middle section of the oven. Preheat the oven to 450°F (230°C). Set a V-shaped rack inside a roasting pan.

Once ready to cook, remove the turkey from the yogurt marinade and wipe off as much as possible. Squeeze out as much marinade as possible from underneath the turkey skin as well.

Grab the turkey by the legs and carefully transfer to the prepared roasting pan with the breast side up. With your hands, rub about a third of the tandoori ghee over the bird, then rub another third underneath the skin. Reserve the remaining ghee for basting the turkey.

Stuff the cavity with the lemons, garlic, ginger, and cilantro. Tuck the wings underneath the turkey, then tie the legs together with kitchen twine, wrapping around the bird to secure.

Pour 3 cups of chicken stock into the bottom of the roasting pan.

Roast the turkey for 30 minutes, rotating halfway, until the skin is mostly golden brown. While the turkey roasts, melt the remaining third of tandoori ghee in a small saucepan over low heat, or in a small bowl in the microwave.

After roasting for 30 minutes, baste the turkey with the melted ghee. Reduce the oven temperature to 300°F (150°C). If the bottom of the pan looks dry, pour in 1–2 more cups of stock. Continue roasting, basting and rotating the turkey every 30 minutes, until a meat thermometer inserted in the thickest part of the leg reaches 165°F (75°C), 120–150 minutes more. The skin should be shiny, crisp, and golden brown–if the skin begins to get too dark, lightly tend the bird with aluminum foil. Remove the turkey from the oven and baste once more. Let rest for 30–60 minutes. Reserve the drippings, discarding the fat, for making the gravy.

Make the tandoori gravy: Add the reserved ¼ cup tandoori ghee to a medium saucepan over medium heat. Add the flour and cook, whisking frequently, for 3–5 minutes, until the roux is darker in color and smells fragrant and toasted. Add 1 tablespoon of the tandoori spice blend and whisk to combine, letting toast for another minute, until fragrant. Gradually whisk in the turkey drippings (adding chicken stock as needed for a total of 3 cups). Bring to a boil, then reduce the heat to medium-low and simmer for 10–15 minutes, until thickened slightly. Remove the gravy from heat.

To serve, set the whole turkey in the center of a large platter for a classic presentation, or carve the bird and arrange the cut pieces on the platter and garnish with cilantro and quartered limes. Serve immediately with the hot gravy alongside, as well as any traditional tandoori sides of choice.

Oxtail Beignets

What You Need -

for 4 servings

OXTAIL STEW

2 teaspoons freshly ground black pepper

1 tablespoon kosher salt

2 teaspoons McCormick® Garlic Powder

2 teaspoons McCormick® Onion Powder

2 teaspoons ground allspice

3 tablespoons dark brown sugar

2 ½ lb oxtail(1.2 kg), cleaned

2 tablespoons vegetable oil, divided

1 tablespoon soy sauce

1 tablespoon worcestershire sauce

2 teaspoons browning sauce

5 cloves garlic, smashed

½ medium yellow onion, chopped

1 cup celery(125 g), chopped

1 cup carrot(150 g), chopped

1 cup scallions(40 g), chopped

1 scotch bonnet pepper

1 teaspoon whole allspice berry

2 bay leaves, dried

4 sprigs fresh thyme

1 teaspoon beef bouillon powder

1 tablespoon ketchup

3 cups beef broth(720 mL)

SPICE MIXTURE

2 tablespoons lightly dried parsley

½ teaspoon allspice, ground

½ tablespoon McCormick® Paprika

½ teaspoon kosher salt

BEIGNETS

2 qt peanut oil(1.9 kg), for frying

all purpose flour, for dusting

1 batch Tasty's Beignet

Method

Prepare the oxtails: In a small bowl, mix together the black pepper, salt, garlic powder, onion powder, ground allspice, and brown sugar.

Place the oxtails in a large bowl and rub all over with the spice blend. Cover with plastic wrap and marinate in the refrigerator for at least 45 minutes, or overnight.

After marinating, remove the oxtails from the refrigerator. Set the Instant Pot to high sauté.

While the Instant Pot is heating, whisk together the soy sauce, Worcestershire sauce, and browning sauce in a small bowl. Massage the sauce mixture into the oxtails until well coated on all sides.

Heat 1 tablespoon of vegetable oil in the Instant Pot until shimmering, then add the oxtails and brown on all sides, being careful not to burn, about 2 minutes per side. Remove the oxtails from the pot and transfer to a clean bowl.

Add the remaining tablespoon of vegetable oil to the Instant Pot. When the oil is shimmering, add the garlic, onion, celery, and carrots. Cook until the vegetables are translucent, stirring occasionally, 2–3 minutes. Add the scallions, habanero pepper, allspice berries, bay leaves, thyme, bouillon powder, and ketchup and cook for another 2 minutes, until well combined.

Return the oxtails to the pot, then pour in the beef broth. Secure the lid of the Instant Pot and seal the vent. Set to pressure cook on high for 62 minutes.

Once the Instant Pot timer goes off, allow the pressure to naturally release. Remove the lid and transfer the oxtails to a cutting board. Remove the meat from the bones and transfer the meat to a fine-mesh strainer set over a small bowl to catch any remaining liquid. Pour the remaining liquid in the pot, along with the meat drippings, through the strainer into a medium bowl. Chill in the refrigerator for 20–30 minutes, until the fat rises to the surface. Skim off the fat and discard.

Transfer the skimmed broth to a 2-quart pot. Cook over medium-high heat until reduced by half, 15–20 minutes. Cover to keep warm until ready to serve, then transfer to a small bowl for dipping.

Make the spice mixture: Add the dried parsley, allspice, paprika, and salt until to a spice grinder and grind into a fine powder, about 10–12 pulses. Transfer to a small bowl.

Heat the peanut oil in a 4-quart pot over medium-high heat until the temperature reaches 350°F (180°C). Set a wire rack over a baking sheet.

After the beignet dough has proofed, roll out on a lightly floured surface to about ¼ inch thick. Trim the edges, then cut into about 16 3-inch squares.

Roll each dough square out into a rectangle. Scoop 1 tablespoon of the oxtail meat onto one side of each rectangle, leaving space around the edges. Fold the other side of the beignet over the meat and press the edges together to seal.

Working in batches of 3–4, fry the beignets in the hot oil for 2–3 minutes on each side, until light golden brown. Transfer to the wire rack to drain and immediately sprinkle the spice mix on top.

Place the beignets on a platter, top with the spice mix, and serve with the reduced broth for dipping.

Enjoy!

Malaysian Chicken Curry Laksa (Laksa Lemak)

What You Need -

for 2 servings

LAKSA PASTE

8 dried red chilies

2 tablespoons dried shrimp

2 tablespoons raw cashews

1 tablespoon whole coriander seeds

½ teaspoon whole cumin seeds

1 tablespoon shrimp paste

1 piece fresh ginger, chopped

1 piece fresh galangal, chopped

1 piece fresh turmeric, chopped

6 cloves garlic, peeled

6 Thai red chiles, stemmed

4 shallots, chopped

2 stalks lemongrass, white parts only

1 tablespoon oriental curry powder

2 tablespoons fresh cilantro, stems an roots

¼ cup vegetable oil(60 mL)

CURRY

1 tablespoon kosher salt, plus more for boiling

7 oz egg noodle, or wide rice vermicelli

2 tablespoons vegetable oil

1 teaspoon fresh ginger, minced

1 teaspoon garlic, minced

½ teaspoon Thai red chiles, minced

1 teaspoon lemongrass, white part only, minced

2 boneless, skinless chicken thighs, sliced

3 long beans, cut into 4-6 inches (10-15 cm)

2 cups chicken stock(480 mL)

1 can full fat coconut milk

6 fresh tofus, deep fried

6 fish cakes, deep-fried (optional)

8 slices rice cake, optional

1 ½ teaspoons palm sugar, plus more to taste

2 limes, plus more to taste

FOR GARNISH

fresh cilantro leaf, chopped, small bunch

fresh mint leaf, chopped

2 lime wedges

2 hard boiled eggs, halved lengthwise

2 Thai red chiles, sliced

1 tablespoon sambal oelek, such as Huy Fong

Method

Make the laksa paste: In a food processor, combine the dried red chiles, dried shrimp, cashews, coriander seeds, and cumin seeds and grind into a powder. Add the shrimp paste, ginger, galangal, turmeric, garlic, Thai red chiles, shallots, lemongrass, curry powder, cilantro stems and roots, and vegetable oil and grind into a smooth paste, about 3 minutes. Set aside until ready to use. The laksa paste will keep in an airtight container in the refrigerator for up to one week. Pour a bit of oil over the top to cover the sauce before storing.

Make the curry: Bring a large pot of salted water to a boil. Add the noodles and cook according to the package instructions, then drain and set aside.

Heat the vegetable oil in a large, heavy-bottomed pan over medium heat. Add the ginger and garlic and sauté for 1–2 minutes, until fragrant, then add the Thai red chiles and lemongrass and sauté for 2 minutes, until the lemongrass softens a bit. Add the laksa paste and sauté for 2–3 minutes, until the oil starts to separate. Add the chicken thighs and cook for 3–4 minutes, until about halfway cooked. Add the long beans and sauté for 2 minutes, until the beans soften a bit.

Add the chicken stock and coconut milk. Bring to a boil, then remove the pot from the heat.

Add the tofu, fish cakes and rice cakes, if using, 1 tablespoon salt, the palm sugar, and lime juice and stir to incorporate. Season the curry with more salt, lime juice, or palm sugar, if desired.

Divide the cooked noodles between 2 deep bowls. Ladle the curry sauce over the noodles, then use tongs to distribute the chicken, tofu puffs, fish cakes, rice cakes, and long beans on top. Garnish with the cilantro, mint, lime wedges, hard-boiled eggs, Thai red chiles, and sambal oelek.

Enjoy!

Torta Ahogada

What You Need -

for 4 servings

CARNITAS

3 tablespoons kosher salt

1 tablespoon freshly ground black pepper

1 tablespoon dried mexican oregano

1 tablespoon Mccormick® ground cumin

4 lb boneless, skinless pork butt(1.7 kg)

3 oranges

8 cloves garlic, peeled and smashed

1 medium yellow onion, peeled and quartered
with stem still attached

TOMATO SALSA

1 tablespoon canola oil

½ lb roma tomato(225 g), quartered

½ large yellow onion, diced

1 clove garlic, minced

1 tablespoon kosher salt

½ tablespoon freshly ground black pepper

1 ½ teaspoons dried mexican oregano

1 ½ teaspoons margarine

2 cups chicken stock(480 mL)

RED ONION ESCABECHE

2 limes, juiced

1 tablespoon kosher salt

1 teaspoon dried mexican oregano, crushed

½ medium red onion, thinly sliced

SPICY SALSA

10 whole japones chiles

1 tablespoon canola oil

½ lb roma tomato(225 g), quartered

½ large yellow onion, diced

3 cloves garlic, minced

2 tablespoons kosher salt

½ teaspoon Mccormick® ground cumin

2 tablespoons distilled white vinegar

ASSEMBLY

4 birotes

lime wedge

Method

Make the carnitas: Preheat the oven to 275°F (135°C).

In a small bowl, whisk together the salt, pepper, oregano, and cumin.

Set the pork butt on a rimmed baking sheet and pat try with paper towels. Rub the spice mixture over the pork butt to cover completely.

Cut the oranges in half and juice. Set the juice aside.

Spread the orange rinds, garlic, and onion in an even layer on the bottom of a heavy-bottomed pot. Place the pork butt on top and pour the orange juice over. Cover the pot with a lid or 2 layers of heavy-duty aluminum foil and cook in the oven until the pork is tender and can be shredded with a fork, about 8 hours.

Make the tomato salsa: Heat the canola oil in a large pan over medium heat. When the oil begins to shimmer, add the tomatoes, onion, and garlic and sauté until the onion begins to caramelize, about 3 minutes. Add the salt, pepper, oregano, and margarine and continue cooking until fragrant, about 2 minutes. Add the chicken stock, increase the heat to medium-high, and bring to a simmer. Continue cooking until the vegetables are soft, about 15 minutes.

Transfer the mixture to a blender and blend on medium-high speed until completely smooth.

Pour the salsa back into the pan and cook over medium-low heat until thickened, about 10 minutes. Rinse out the blender basin.

Make the red onion escabeche: In a medium bowl, whisk together the lime juice, salt, and oregano. Add the onion and toss to coat. Let sit for at least 15 minutes, or cover and refrigerate for up to 1 week.

Make the spicy salsa: In a large pan over medium-high heat, toast the Japones chiles until fragrant, about 2 minutes. Remove the chiles from the pan and set aside.

Heat the canola oil in the same pan over medium heat. When the oil begins to shimmer, add the tomatoes, onion, and garlic and sauté until the onion begins to caramelize, about 3 minutes. Add the salt and cumin and continue cooking until the tomatoes are tender, about 8 minutes.

Transfer the mixture to the blender. Add the toasted chiles and distilled white vinegar and blend on medium-high speed until smooth.

Assemble the tortas: Use a fork to shred the carnitas.

Cut the birotes down the middle, leaving one long side intact, like a hot dog bun. Fill the rolls with carnitas and pour the tomato salsa on top. Serve with the spicy salsa, escabeche, and lime wedges.

Enjoy!

Peanut Butter & Jelly Spiders

What You Need -

for 1 spider

2 slices whole grain bread

nut butter, to taste

jelly, to taste

8 pretzel sticks

2 raisins

Method

Using the lid of a wide mouth mason jar, carve out rounds into both slices of bread, remove the crusts.

Spread peanut butter evenly across one side of one of the rounds and spread jelly evenly across one side of the other round.

Place peanut butter round and jelly round together to create the "body" of the spider.

Place 4 pretzel sticks into the left side of the sandwich and 4 pretzel sticks into the right side, creating the "spider legs."

Place raisins on the sandwich to create the "eyes."

Enjoy!

Meal Prep Pesto Chicken Pasta

What You Need -

for 4 servings

1 tablespoon oil

salt, to taste

1 lb large chicken breast(455 g), cooked and diced

2 cups asparagus(250 g), cut into 1 1/2-in/38-mm pieces

10 oz cherry tomatoes(285 g), halved

⅔ cup pesto(150 g)

2 cups whole wheat penne(200 g), measured dry

parsley, for garnish

Method

Heat the oil in a large nonstick skillet. Toss in the asparagus, season with a bit of salt, and sautée until the begin to soften, about 3 minutes.

Pour on the pesto, pasta, and chicken and stir to combine.

Toss in the cherry tomatoes and give everything a stir to combine and warm through.

Distribute pasta mixture evenly between 4 tupperware containers.

Top with parsley for garnish.

Can be refrigerated up to 4 days.

Enjoy!

NUTRITIOUS DISHES FOR EVENING MEALS

One-Pot Pesto Chicken Pasta

What You Need -

for 4 servings

1 lb boneless, skinless chicken tenders(455 g)

1 tablespoon olive oil

3 cloves garlic

16 fl oz low-sodium chicken broth

4 oz sun-dried tomatoes(110 g), drained

8 oz whole wheat pasta(225 g)

¼ teaspoon salt

¼ teaspoon red pepper flakes

3 oz baby spinach(85 g)

PESTO

1 clove garlic

4 oz fresh basil(110 g), roughly chopped

¼ teaspoon salt

¼ teaspoon black pepper

2 tablespoons walnuts

3 oz olive oil(90 mL)

4 tablespoons fresh parmesan cheese

Method

For the pesto, add garlic, basil, salt, pepper, and walnuts into the bowl of a food processor.

Turn on the food processor and slowly add the olive oil in a steady stream and puree thoroughly.

Add the parmesan and pulse to incorporate. Set aside.

In a large pot, heat olive oil on medium-high heat. Season chicken and brown on both sides. Cook thoroughly for 8-10 minutes. Remove chicken from pan and set aside.

Sauté garlic for 1-2 minutes, or until fragrant. Add the chicken broth, sun-dried tomatoes, pasta, salt, and red pepper flakes and mix until combined. Cover.

Bring liquid to a boil. Reduce heat and simmer for 10-15 minutes, or until pasta is al dente.

Add spinach and stir until wilted.

Add cooked chicken and pesto.

Serve immediately.

Enjoy!

Crunchy Avocado Tuna Wraps

What You Need -

for 4 servings

5 oz tuna(140 g), 2 cans, drained

1 large avocado, diced

1 cup carrot(110 g), finely chopped

2 ribs celery, finely chopped

¼ cup red onion(35 g), finely chopped

¼ cup dijon mustard(60 g)

1 tablespoon lemon juice

½ teaspoon garlic powder

salt, to taste

pepper, to taste

4 whole wheat tortillas

4 leaves green leaf lettuce

1 cup cherry tomatoes(200 g), halved

Method

In a large bowl, add the tuna and avocado. Use a fork to smash the avocado and tuna together.

Add the carrots, celery, red onion, Dijon mustard, lemon juice, garlic powder, salt, and pepper. Stir to combine.

Lay a tortilla flat on a plate. Lay a lettuce leaf on the tortilla. Scoop ¼ of the tuna mixture into the center of the lettuce and spread down the middle. Top with cherry tomatoes and carefully roll the the tortilla to create a wrap. Repeat with the remaining ingredients.

Enjoy!

One-Pan Chicken Adobo

What You Need -

for 4 servings

2 lb chicken(910 g)

3 dried bay leaves

5 tablespoons soy sauce

2 tablespoons vinegar

3 garlics, crushed

1 cup water(240 mL)

¼ cup cooking oil(60 mL)

1 tablespoon white sugar

salt, to taste

whole peppercorn

Method

In a container or a plastic food bag, combine soy sauce and garlic then marinade the chicken for 30 minutes.

Place a medium pan on medium heat and add oil, once the oil is hot put the marinated chicken and brown (about five minutes).

Pour in the remaining marinade and add water, then bring to a boil.

Add the dried bay leaves and whole peppercorn. Simmer for 30 minutes or until the chicken is tender.

Add the vinegar, stir and simmer for 10 more minutes.

Add the sugar, salt, and stir. Then remove from heat.

Enjoy!

The Best Homemade Pizza

What You Need -

for 16 servings

2 ½ cups warm water(600 mL)

1 teaspoon sugar

2 teaspoons active dry yeast

7 cups all-purpose flour(875 g), plus more for dusting

6 tablespoons extra virgin olive oil, plus more for greasing

1 ½ teaspoons kosher salt

¼ cup semolina flour(30 g)

OPTIONAL TOPPINGS

TOMATO SAUCE

28 oz canned whole tomatoes(795 g)

1 tablespoon kosher salt

MARGHERITA

tomato sauce

fresh mozzarella cheese, torn into small pieces

fresh basil leaf

TASTY'S BIANCA

extra virgin olive oil

fresh mozzarella cheese, torn into small pieces

ricotta cheese

fresh basil pesto

dried oregano

PEPPERONI

tomato sauce

fresh mozzarella cheese, torn into small pieces

spicy pepperoni slice

freshly grated parmesan cheese

Method

"Bloom" the yeast by sprinkling the sugar and yeast in the warm water. Let sit for 10 minutes, until bubbles form on the surface.

In a large bowl, combine the flour and salt. Make a well in the middle and add the olive oil and bloomed yeast mixture. Using a spoon, mix until a shaggy dough begins to form.

Once the flour is mostly hydrated, turn the dough out onto a clean work surface and knead for 10-15 minutes. The dough should be soft, smooth, and bouncy. Form the dough into a taut round.

Grease a clean, large bowl with olive oil and place the dough inside, turning to coat with the oil. Cover with plastic wrap. Let rise for at least an hour, or up to 24 hours.

Punch down the dough and turn it out onto a lightly floured work surface. Knead for another minute or so, then cut into 4 equal portions and shape into rounds.

Lightly flour the dough, then cover with a kitchen towel and let rest for another 30 minutes to an hour while you prepare the sauce and any other ingredients.

Preheat the oven as high as your oven will allow, between 450-500°F (230-260°C). Place a pizza stone, heavy baking sheet (turn upside down so the surface is flat), or cast iron skillet in the oven.

Meanwhile, make the tomato sauce: Add the salt to the can of tomatoes and puree with an immersion blender, or transfer to a blender or food processor, and puree until smooth.

Once the dough has rested, take a portion and start by poking the surface with your fingertips, until bubbles form and do not deflate.

Then, stretch and press the dough into a thin round. Make it thinner than you think it should be, as it will slightly shrink and puff up during baking.

Sprinkle semolina onto an upside down baking sheet and place the stretched crust onto it. Add the sauce and ingredients of your choice.

Slide the pizza onto the preheated pizza stone or pan. Bake for 15 minutes, or until the crust and cheese are golden brown.

Add any garnish of your preference.

Nutrition Calories: 1691 Fat: 65 grams Carbs: 211 grams Fiber: 12 grams Sugars: 60 grams Protein: 65 grams

Enjoy!

Pesto Garden Pasta For The Whole Family

What You Need -

for 6 servings

PESTO SAUCE

2 cups fresh basil leaves(80 g)

½ cup olive oil(120 mL)

½ cup grated parmesan cheese(55 g)

1 tablespoon almond butter

1 tablespoon lemon juice

2 cloves garlic, smashed

2 teaspoons lemon zest

kosher salt, to taste

pepper, to taste

PASTA

kosher salt, to taste

4 cups pasta(800 g), short, such as farfalle or penne

1 cup grape tomato(200 g), halved

1 cup yellow cherry tomato(200 g), halved

¼ cup red onion(35 g), sliced

8 oz mozzarella ball(225 g), drained

Method

Add the basil, olive oil, Parmesan, almond butter, lemon juice, garlic, lemon zest, salt, and pepper to a blender. Blend until smooth and set aside.

Cook the pasta according to the package instructions.

Drain and transfer the pasta to a large serving bowl.

Add the grape tomatoes, yellow tomatoes, red onion, and mozzarella balls to the pasta.

Pour the pesto sauce over the pasta.

Toss the ingredients together.

Serve warm in a bowl.

Enjoy!

Pumpkin Sage Pasta

What You Need -

for 4 servings

1 tablespoon cooking oil, of preference

½ white onion, diced

2 cloves garlic, minced

½ teaspoon red pepper flakes, optional

½ teaspoon dried sage

1 ½ cups almond milk(360 mL)

15 oz pumpkin puree(425 g)

1 teaspoon salt

1 teaspoon pepper

¼ teaspoon nutmeg

½ box whole wheat pasta, cooked

Method

Heat the oil in a medium pot over medium heat. Add the onion, garlic, red pepper flakes, and dried sage and cook until onions are translucent, stirring occasionally.

Add the almond milk, pumpkin puree, salt, pepper, and nutmeg. Stir until a smooth, creamy sauce forms. Heat through.

Add the cooked pasta and and stir to coat.

Serve warm.

Enjoy!

Country Fried Steak And Gravy

What You Need -

for 4 servings

8 oz cube steak(225 g), 4 steaks, 8 oz (225 g) each

1 ½ teaspoons kosher salt, plus more to taste

1 teaspoon black pepper, plus more to taste

2 large eggs

2 ¾ cups whole milk(660 mL), divided

1 ½ cups all-purpose flour(190 g), divided, plus

3 tablespoons

1 teaspoon garlic powder

1 teaspoon onion powder

1 teaspoon paprika

1 cup vegetable oil(240 mL)

3 tablespoons unsalted butter

½ cup heavy cream(120 mL)

Method

Preheat the oven to 225°F (110°C).

Set a steak in the center of a cutting board and cover with a piece of plastic wrap. Using a meat mallet, pound the steak evenly to ¼-inch

(½ cm) thick. Season with salt and pepper on both sides. Repeat with the remaining meat.

In a wide, shallow dish, whisk together the eggs and 1 cup (240 ml) of milk. In a separate shallow dish, mix together the 1 ½ cups (190 g) of flour, pepper, salt, garlic powder, onion powder, and paprika.

Dredge the steaks in the flour mixture, then dip in the egg mixture, letting any excess egg drip off. Coat again in the flour mixture. Set aside for 10-15 minutes, until the coating has dried out a bit.

Meanwhile, heat the oil in a 10-inch (25.5 cm) pan over medium-high heat until it reaches 375°F (190°C).

Fry the steaks, 2 at a time, for 3 minutes, until golden brown and crispy. Flip and cook on the other side for 3 minutes more, until golden brown and cooked through when the internal temperature reaches 155°-165°F (170°-175°C). Transfer the steaks to a paper towel-lined plate or baking sheet and immediately season with salt. Once all of the steaks are done frying, transfer to the oven while you prepare the gravy.

Pour the hot oil into a heatproof bowl and let cool before discarding. 9. Leave any browned bits in the pan.

In the same pan, without wiping it out, melt the butter over medium heat. Add the remaining 3 tablespoons of flour, whisking to incorporate. Cook for 2-3 minutes, until the roux is a light brown color. Add the heavy cream and remaining milk. Bring to a simmer and cook, whisking constantly, until thickened, 5-7 minutes. Season with salt and pepper.

Ladle the gravy over the steaks and serve with your favorite side dishes.

Enjoy!

Baked Chicken Parmesan

What You Need -

for 2 servings

2 chicken breasts

2 eggs, beaten

1 ball fresh mozzarella cheese, thinly sliced

1 jar marinara sauce, heated

whole wheat pasta

fresh basil, for garnish

BREADING

½ cup panko bread crumbs(25 g)

½ cup parmesan cheese(55 g)

1 tablespoon fresh basil

½ teaspoon garlic powder

2 teaspoons dried oregano

¼ teaspoon salt

¼ teaspoon black pepper

Method

Preheat oven to 425°F (215°C).

In a medium bowl, combine the panko, parmesan cheese, basil, garlic powder, oregano, salt, and pepper.

Beat the 2 eggs in a shallow dish. Dredge the chicken in the egg wash, then coat with the bread crumb mixture.

Transfer the breaded chicken breasts to a greased roasting pan. Top the chicken with 2 small slices of mozzarella.

Bake for 20-25 min, until the cheese and bread crumbs have turned golden brown and the chicken is cooked through, or until it has reached an internal temperature of 165°F (73°C).

Serve with whole wheat spaghetti, marinara sauce, and a sprinkle of fresh basil.

Enjoy!

Tuna Burgers

What You Need -

for 4 servings

15 oz tuna(425 g), canned, drained

1 tablespoon olive oil, plus more for cooking

¾ cup panko bread crumbs(35 g)

1 tablespoon dried parsley

2 teaspoons fresh chives, minced

1 tablespoon garlic, minced

½ teaspoon salt

½ teaspoon pepper

1 teaspoon paprika

1 large egg, beaten

whole wheat burger bun, for serving

Method

Combine the tuna, olive oil, panko, parsley, chives, garlic, salt, pepper, paprika, and egg in a large bowl until evenly mixed.

Divide the mixture into 4 portions and form patties with your hands.

Heat a drizzle of olive oil in a large skillet over medium-high heat.

Place the patties in the pan and cook for 3-5 minutes on each side, until golden brown.

Serve on whole wheat buns with your preferred toppings.

Enjoy!

BBQ Chicken Pita Pizza

What You Need -

for 1 serving

1 cup rotisserie chicken(125 g), shredded

4 tablespoons BBQ sauce(30 g), divided

1 whole wheat pita bread

1 handful shredded mozzarella cheese

1 handful red onion, sliced

fresh cilantro, for garnish

Method

Preheat the oven to 350°F (180°C). Line a baking sheet with parchment paper.

In a medium bowl, toss the chicken with 2 tablespoons of BBQ sauce until well-coated.

Place the pita bread on the prepared baking sheet and spread the remaining 2 tablespoons of BBQ sauce on top. Scatter the chicken over the pita, then top with shredded mozzarella and red onion.

Bake for 15-20 minutes, or until the cheese is melted and the chicken is heated through.

Garnish with fresh cilantro, then slice and serve.

Enjoy!

Easy Slow Cooker Mozzarella-Stuffed Meatballs And Sauce

What You Need -

for 14 meatballs

SAUCE

7 cups crushed tomato(1.4 kg)

⅓ cup onion(50 g), chopped

2 cloves garlic, crushed

2 teaspoons dried basil

1 teaspoon dried oregano

½ teaspoon pepper

½ teaspoon salt

MEATBALLS

1 lb beef(455 g)

1 lb mild sausage(455 g)

1 cup breadcrumb(115 g)

⅓ cup onion(50 g), chopped

¼ cup parmesan cheese(25 g)

1 teaspoon onion powder

1 teaspoon garlic powder

1 teaspoon dried thyme

1 teaspoon dried oregano

½ teaspoon salt

½ teaspoon pepper

2 eggs

4 sticks mozzarella cheese, cut into 4-5 even pieces each

½ cup whole milk

½ cup parsley

Method

Combine all sauce ingredients in slow cooker and stir. Set to high and cover while making meatballs, or for 30 minutes. (Or use pre-made/canned sauce.)

Combine all meatball ingredients except the mozzarella in a large bowl. Using your hands, mix until fully combined.

Take a golf ball sized piece of the ground beef mixture and place a piece of mozzarella in the middle. Press meat around the piece of cheese, fully enclosing it. Repeat until all meat is used.

Place meatballs in slow cooker and submerge in sauce.

Cover and cook on high for 2-2½ hours, or until meat is fully cooked.

Serve by itself or over pasta.

Enjoy!

Pulled Pork-Stuffed Milk Buns

What You Need -

for 9 servings

STARTER

3 tablespoons water

3 tablespoons whole milk

2 tablespoons bread flour

DOUGH

3 ¼ cups bread flour(410 g), divided

¼ cup sugar(50 g)

1 teaspoon salt

1 tablespoon instant yeast

1 cup whole milk(240 mL), warm to the touch

¼ cup unsalted butter(60 g), 1/2 stick, melted

1 large egg

1 tablespoon vegetable oil

1 ¼ cups pulled pork(310 g)

1 large egg, mixed with 1 tablespoon milk

Method

Make the starter: In a small pot over low heat, combine the water, milk, and flour. Stir continuously until a loose paste forms. Remove the pot from the heat and transfer the mixture to a small bowl. Cover with plastic wrap, pressing it directly onto the surface of the starter, and refrigerate for 1 hour, or until cool.

Make the dough: In a large bowl, add 2½ cups (300 g) of flour, the sugar, salt, and yeast, and whisk to combine.

In a large measuring cup, whisk together the milk, egg, butter, and chilled starter mixture.

Gradually pour the milk mixture into the bowl of dry ingredients, using your hands to combine. The dough will be very sticky at this point. If the dough is too wet to knead, gradually add ¾ cup (90 g) of flour, a few tablespoons at a time, until you can knead the dough into a loose ball. Continue to knead the dough for 20 minutes.

Cover your hands with the vegetable oil and form the dough into a taut ball. Place the dough into a clean large bowl. Cover with a towel and let rise in a warm place until doubled in size, 60-90 minutes.

Transfer the dough to a clean surface and press out to a 9-inch (23 cm) square. Divide the dough into 9 equal squares.

Flatten a portion of dough into a circle. Place 2 tablespoons of pulled pork in the center. Pinch the edges of the dough together to seal. Gently roll the dough into a ball and place in a greased 9-inch (23 cm) square baking dish. Repeat with the remaining dough. Cover with a towel and let rise for 45 minutes.

Preheat the oven to 350°F (180°C).

Brush the buns with the egg and milk mixture.

Bake the buns for 25 minutes, or until golden brown.

Let the buns sit in the pan for 10 minutes.

Invert the buns onto a serving plate, and pull apart.

Enjoy!

Healthy Veggie Curry With Garlic Naan

What You Need -

for 8 servings

RICE

2 cups white rice(400 g), rinsed

4 cups water(960 g)

1 tablespoon coconut oil, melted

salt, to taste

CURRY

¼ cup vegetable oil(60 mL), divided

2 small yellow onions, diced

2 cups idaho potato(450 g), cubed

1 tablespoon tomato paste

2 tablespoons fresh ginger, minced

3 cloves garlic, minced

1 ½ teaspoons garam masala

2 tablespoons curry powder

1 head cauliflower, cut into small florets

15 oz diced tomato(425 g), 1 can

15 oz chickpeas(425 g), 1 can, drained

1 ¼ cups water(360 mL)

salt, to taste

¾ cup coconut milk(180 mL)

1 ¼ cups frozen peas(190 g)

GARLIC NAAN

2 cups all-purpose flour(250 g)

1 teaspoon salt

1 teaspoon baking powder

1 teaspoon sugar

2 tablespoons ghee, melted, divided, plus more
as needed

4 tablespoons whole-fat yogurt

2 tablespoons skim milk

6 tablespoons water

1 clove garlic, minced

Method

In a medium pot, combine the rice, water,
coconut oil, and salt. Bring to a boil, then cover
and simmer over low heat for 15-20 minutes,

until the water is absorbed. Once finished cooking, remove the rice from the heat and fluff.

Heat 3 tablespoons of vegetable oil in a large Dutch oven over medium-high heat until shimmering. Add the onions and potatoes and cook, stirring occasionally, until the onions are caramelized and potatoes are golden brown around the edges, about 10 minutes.

Reduce the heat to medium. Add the remaining tablespoon of oil, the tomato paste, ginger, and garlic. Cook, stirring constantly, until fragrant, about 30 seconds. Add the garam masala and curry powder and cook, stirring constantly, about 1 minute longer.

Add cauliflower and cook, stirring constantly, until the spices coat the florets, about 2 minutes longer.

Add the tomatoes, chickpeas, water, and salt and stir to combine. Increase the heat to medium-high and bring the mixture to a boil. Reduce the heat to medium. Simmer, stirring occasionally, until the vegetables are tender, 10-15 minutes.

Stir in the coconut milk and frozen peas. Cook until heated through, about 2 minutes longer. Remove from the heat.

Meanwhile, in a large bowl, stir together the flour, salt, baking powder, and sugar. Create a well in the middle of the dry ingredients and pour in 1 tablespoon of melted ghee, the yogurt, skim milk, and a bit of the water. Mix until combined, adding more water as needed until the dough comes together.

Transfer the dough to a lightly floured surface and knead until no longer sticky, then shape into a ball and divide into quarters. Roll out the dough portions to ¼ inch (6 mm) thick.

In a small bowl, combine the remaining tablespoon of melted ghee with the garlic.

Heat a bit of ghee in a medium nonstick pan over medium-high heat. Add a dough round and brush with the ghee and garlic mixture. Cook for 3-4 minutes, until the dough bubbles up and forms a nice brown crust, then flip and cook on the other side. Repeat with the remaining dough.

Serve the curry over the rice with the naan on the side.

Enjoy!

Copycat Campfire Chicken

What You Need -

for 2 servings

1 tablespoon paprika

2 teaspoons onion powder

2 teaspoons salt

1 teaspoon garlic powder

1 teaspoon dried rosemary

1 teaspoon black pepper

1 teaspoon dried oregano

1 whole chicken, quartered

2 carrots, cut into thirds

3 red skin potatoes, halved

1 ear corn, quartered

1 tablespoon olive oil

1 tablespoon butter

5 sprigs fresh thyme

Method

Combine paprika, onion powder, salt, garlic powder, rosemary, pepper, and oregano in a small bowl and mix well. Reserve 1 tablespoon of the spice mix and set aside.

In a large ziplock bag, place the quartered chicken and spice mix. Marinate for 1 hour or overnight.

Preheat the oven to 400°F (200°C).

Add the carrots, potatoes, and corn to a bowl and drizzle with oil and remaining 1 tablespoon of spice mix and toss until thoroughly coated.

Heat a large pan with oil over high heat. Add the chicken pieces and cook until golden brown on both side. Set aside.

Place the chicken and veggies on a sheet of aluminium foil. Top with butter and thyme. Fold the foil over the chicken and vegetables and cinch the edge so that no air can escape.

Bake for 45 minutes, or chicken is completely cooked.

Enjoy!

Honey Mustard Glazed Ham

What You Need -

for 12 servings

onion, chopped

10 cloves garlic, peeled

¼ cup apple cider vinegar(60 mL)

¼ cup stone ground mustard(60 g)

1 cup orange juice(240 mL)

10 whole cloves

10 lb picnic ham(4 ½ kg), cured

½ cup honey(170 g)

½ cup dijon mustard(125 g)

1 tablespoon worcestershire sauce

1 cup brown sugar(220 g)

Method

Preheat oven to 400°F (200°C).

Add the chopped onion, garlic cloves, apple cider vinegar, mustard, orange juice, and cloves to a large roasting pan, stirring to combine.

Place the ham on the roasting rack over the liquid.

Trim off tough outer skin, then score the remaining fat in a crosshatch pattern. Cover the entire roasting rack with aluminum foil and bake for 1 hour.

Remove the ham from the oven, and remove the foil. Baste the ham with the liquid, then remove the rack from the roasting pan and set aside.

Remove all the whole cloves from the remaining liquid in the pan. Pour the remaining liquid into a pot, along with the honey, Dijon mustard, Worcestershire sauce, and brown sugar. Whisk to combine.

Bring the mixture to a boil over medium high heat, then simmer until thick and reduced, about 10 minutes.

Brush the glaze on to the ham then transfer back to the roasting rack.

Bake the ham for 30-45 minutes, or until the glaze is caramelized and the ham reaches 145°F (65°C).

Slice the ham, and serve.

Enjoy!

Homemade Chicken Shawarma

What You Need -

for 4 servings

2 ½ lb boneless, skinless chicken thighs(1.1 kg), trimmed

MARINADE

1 teaspoon cumin

1 teaspoon ground cardamom

1 tablespoon paprika

½ teaspoon cinnamon

1 teaspoon turmeric

1 teaspoon garlic powder

1 tablespoon sumac

¼ teaspoon cayenne

1 tablespoon kosher salt

1 teaspoon fresh ground black pepper

4 tablespoons olive oil

1 tablespoon fresh lemon juice

3 cloves garlic, sliced

WHITE SAUCE

1 cup whole milk greek yogurt(245 g)

1 tablespoon lemon juice

1 clove garlic, minced

1 teaspoon sumac

⅛ teaspoon cayenne pepper

¼ teaspoon salt

¼ teaspoon black pepper

FOR SERVING

pita bread, warmed

cucumber, sliced

tomato, sliced

pickle

Method

Combine all marinade ingredients in a large bowl and whisk together.

Add the chicken thighs and coat evenly.

Cover and chill for at least 1 hour and up to 12 hours

Prepare the sauce by adding all sauce ingredients to a small bowl. Mix together and chill until ready to serve.

Adjust the oven rack about 6 inches (15 cm) from the top heat source in your oven, then preheat the broiler.

Line a baking sheet with foil and a wire rack.

Place chicken in single layer on prepared wire rack, with the smooth sides down. Broil until chicken is well browned and registers at least 165°F (74°C), about 16-20 minutes. You may need to rotate the sheet pan halfway through if your broiler heats unevenly. Remove and rest the chicken for 5 minutes before handling, and turn off the oven.

While chicken rests, warm your pitas in the still-warm oven for a few minutes.

Slice the chicken into thin strips and transfer to platter.

Serve with sliced cucumbers, tomatoes, pickles, prepared yogurt sauce, and warm pita.

Enjoy!

Lasagna-Stuffed Peppers

What You Need -

for 4 servings

4 bell peppers, various colors

1 onion, chopped

4 cloves garlic, chopped

½ lb ground beef(225 g)

½ lb sweet italian sausage(225 g)

1 teaspoon salt

1 teaspoon pepper

28 oz diced tomato(795 g), 1 can

28 oz tomato sauce(795 g), 1 can

15 oz whole milk ricotta cheese(425 g)

1 cup grated parmesan cheese(110 g)

½ cup fresh basil(20 g), chopped

1 egg

4 lasagna noodles, cooked and quartered

1 cup shredded mozzarella cheese(100 g)

2 tablespoons oil

Method

Preheat oven to 350°F (180°C).

Cut the top off of each pepper and remove the seeds. Transfer to a square baking dish. Bake for 20 minutes, to soften.

Heat 2 tablespoons of oil in a large pot, or dutch oven, over medium high heat. Add the onion and garlic, cook until softened.

Add the ground beef, sausage, salt, and pepper. Cook until the meat has browned on all sides.

Add the diced tomatoes and tomato sauce. Bring the mixture to a light simmer. Simmer for 5-10 minutes, remove from heat and set aside.

In a small bowl, combine ricotta, parmesan, basil, and egg. Mix together with a fork, set aside.

Remove the peppers from the oven, drain any excess water that accumulated inside.

Cut the lasagna noodles into quarters and set aside.

Assemble the lasagna in each pepper. Alternate 2 tablespoons of sauce, 1 lasagna noodle, 2 tablespoons ricotta mixture, and 1 lasagna noodle until the peppers are full. Top with mozzarella cheese.

Bake in preheated oven for 20-25 minutes, until the cheese is melted and slightly browned.

Rest for 10 minutes before serving.

Enjoy!

Chicken Curry Naan Bowls

What You Need -

for 6 servings

RED CHICKEN CURRY

2 tablespoons salt

1 tablespoon ground pepper

1 tablespoon ground cumin

1 tablespoon smoked paprika

1 tablespoon ground turmeric

1 tablespoon coriander

1 teaspoon ground cardamom

1 teaspoon dry mustard

1 teaspoon cayenne

½ teaspoon allspice

3 lb boneless, skinless chicken thighs(1.5 g), cut into 2 in (5 cm) cubes

5 tablespoons full-fat yogurt, divided, plus more for serving

9 cloves garlic, minced, divided

1 tablespoon fresh ginger, minced

3 tablespoons olive oil, plus more as needed

3 carrots, chopped

1 white onion, chopped

1 lb yukon gold potato(455 g), chopped

2 tablespoons tomato paste

28 oz crushed tomatoes(795 g), 1 can

2 cups chicken broth(480 mL)

2 cups basmati rice(460 g), or long-grain jasmine, cooked, for serving

1 fresh cilantro, for serving

Lime wedge, for serving

NAAN BOWLS

½ cup warm water(120 mL)

2 tablespoons sugar

1 tablespoon active dry yeast

4 cups all-purpose flour(500 g), plus more for
dusting

1 teaspoon baking powder

1 teaspoon baking soda

1 tablespoon kosher salt, plus more to taste

1 cup full-fat yogurt(245 g)

1 cup whole milk(240 mL), room temperature

olive oil, for greasing

½ cup unsalted butter(115 g), 1 stick, melted

Method

In a small bowl, combine the salt, pepper, cumin, smoked paprika, turmeric, coriander, cardamom, dry mustard, cayenne, and allspice. Stir to combine.

In a large bowl, add the cubed chicken thighs, 2 tablespoons of yogurt, 4 cloves of minced garlic, the ginger, and half of the spice mixture. Toss the chicken until it is fully coated. Cover the bowl with plastic wrap, and marinate in the fridge for 2 hours or overnight.

Make the naan bowls: In a liquid measuring cup, combine the warm water, sugar, and yeast. Set aside to bloom for 10 minutes.

In the meantime, mix the flour, baking powder, baking soda, and salt together in a large bowl.

To the yeast mixture, add the yogurt and milk. Stir until smooth, then pour into the dry ingredients. Stir to combine, then dump the dough out onto a floured surface and knead with your hands until it forms a smooth, soft ball, about 2 minutes.

Place the dough in a clean large bowl greased with olive oil and cover with a clean kitchen towel or plastic wrap. Let rise at room temperature until doubled in size, about 2 hours.

Heat the olive oil in a large Dutch oven over medium-high heat. Working in batches to avoid overcrowding the pot, cook the marinated chicken on all sides until cooked through and browned, about 20 minutes. Drizzle in more oil, as needed, to prevent the meat from sticking to the bottom of the pot. Transfer the browned meat to a plate as it finishes cooking and set aside.

Add the carrots, onion, potatoes, remaining 5 cloves of minced garlic, and reserved spice mixture, Stir and cook until the vegetables brown slightly and start to soften, 15 minutes.

Stir in the tomato paste and cook until aromatic, about 3 minutes.

Add the crushed tomatoes and chicken broth. Stir to combine. Bring to a simmer.

Add the chicken, stir, and return to a simmer. Cover and cook for 30 minutes, or until the potatoes are tender and the chicken is cooked through.

Stir in the remaining 3 tablespoons of yogurt, then cover and keep warm.

Once the naan dough has risen, dump onto a floured surface, and divide into 6 equal portions. Roll each portion into a ¼-inch (1 /2 cm) thick circle, approximately 10 inches (25 cm) in diameter.

Heat a large cast-iron skillet over medium-high heat. Place a disc of naan dough in the skillet. Cook for about 2 minutes, until the dough puffs up, then flip and cook on the other side until browned, 1 minute. Transfer the naan to a medium bowl and place another bowl on top. Repeat with the rest of the naan dough, stacking bowls between each round. As the naan cools, they will retain the bowl shape.

Brush the naan bowls with warm melted butter.

Fill the naan bowls with the chicken curry and rice. Serve with yogurt, cilantro, and lime wedges.

Enjoy!

Garlic Herb-Crusted Roast Rack Of Lamb

What You Need -

for 8 servings

2 ½ lb rack of lamb(1.1 kg), frenched

salt, to taste

pepper, to taste

5 tablespoons olive oil, divided

8 cloves garlic, peeled and smashed

¾ cup breadcrumb(85 g)

¼ cup fresh flat-leaf parsley(10 g)

1 ½ tablespoons fresh rosemary

½ cup grated parmesan cheese(55 g)

1 ½ tablespoons whole grain dijon mustard

Method

Preheat oven to 400°F (200°C).

Season lamb generously with salt and pepper.

Heat a cast iron over medium high heat.

To the hot pan, add in 4 tablespoons of the the olive oil, along with the lamb and garlic. Sear all sides of the lamb until browned, about 3-4 minutes. Remove browned lamb, and place cooked lamb onto a baking sheet.

Remove garlic and add to food processor with along with the breadcrumbs, parsley, parmesan, rosemary, and 1 tablespoon of olive oil. Pulse until combined. Pour onto a large plate.

Brush the top and sides of the lamb with mustard.

Coat the top and sides of the lamb with the breadcrumb mixture and roast in oven for 20-25 minutes.

Allow to rest before slicing.

Enjoy!

Beet Gnocchi

What You Need -

for 4 servings

1 medium beet, greens trimmed

1 large russet potato

1 large egg

½ cup grated parmesan cheese(55 g), plus more for serving

1 teaspoon kosher salt, plus more for boiling

1 ½ cups whole wheat flour(190 g), plus more for dusting

½ cup salted butter(115 g), 1/2 stick, divided

2 tablespoons fresh sage, chopped, divided

Method

Preheat the oven to 425°F (220°C).

Add the beet to an oven-safe dish and pour in enough water to come ¾ of the way up the beet. Cover the dish tightly with foil and set aside.

Poke the potato all over with a fork and place in the center of a parchment paper-lined baking sheet.

Place both the beet and potato in the oven and roast for 45 minutes, until fork tender. Remove from the oven and let cool until safe to handle.

Gently rub the beet to remove the skin. (If you'd like, wear rubber gloves to protect your hands from being dyed by the beet juice.) Trim any remaining stem from the beet after peeling, then roughly chop.

Transfer the beet to a food processor, along with the egg, Parmesan, and salt. Puree until completely smooth. Set aside.

Peel the skin from potato and grate through the small holes of a box grater, or press through a potato ricer, if you have one.

In a large bowl, combine the potato and the beet mixture. Fold gently to combine, being careful not to over mix.

Add the flour, ½ cup (60 grams) at a time, and fold until the dough comes together. You may not need to use the full 2 cups.

Turn the dough out onto a lightly floured surface and knead gently until a pliable dough is formed that is tender but not sticky when handled. Divide into 8 portions. Roll a dough portion into a ½-inch (1 ¼ cm) thick rope. Cut the rope into 1-inch (2.5 cm) pieces. Repeat with the remaining dough.

If desired, roll each piece of gnocchi over the tines of a fork to create ridges.

Bring a medium pot of well-salted water to a boil over high heat.

Working in batches, drop 8-10 gnocchi into the boiling water and cook until they begin to float. Once they start floating at the surface, let cook for 30 seconds more, then transfer from the water with a slotted spoon to a plate and set aside.

In a medium pan, melt 2 tablespoons of butter until just beginning to bubble. Add 1 tablespoon of sage and half of the gnocchi, to avoid overcrowding the pan. Sauté for about 1 minute per side until the gnocchi are lightly toasted and well coated with butter and sage. Repeat with the remaining butter, sage, and gnocchi.

Serve immediately with Parmesan cheese for garnish.

Enjoy!

NUTRITIOUS DISHES FOR APPETIZERS

Rainbow Veggie Pinwheels

What You Need -

for 4 servings

2 cups chickpeas(330 g), drained and rinsed

1 ½ teaspoons salt

½ teaspoon pepper

½ teaspoon cumin

¼ cup tahini paste(60 g)

2 tablespoons lemon juice

2 tablespoons olive oil

1 package whole wheat tortillas

1 red bell pepper, sliced

2 carrots, sliced

1 yellow bell pepper, sliced

1 cucumber, sliced

¼ shredded purple cabbage

Method

In the bowl of a food processor, add the drained chickpeas, salt, pepper, cumin, tahini paste, lemon juice, and olive oil and pureé until smooth.

On a whole wheat tortilla, spoon on some hummus and add slices of red pepper, carrot, yellow pepper, cucumber, and purple cabbage.

Wrap up the tortilla, and cut into slices to make the pinwheels. Repeat with remaining ingredients.

Slice and serve.

Enjoy!

Chicken And Spinach Pull-Apart Bread

What You Need -

for 15 servings

½ lb rotisserie chicken(225 g)

10 oz cream cheese(285 g), softened

⅔ cup spinach(25 g), cooked and drained

2 cups shredded mozzarella cheese(230 g)

1 teaspoon garlic powder

1 teaspoon pepper

1 teaspoon salt

4 cups flour(500 g)

4 tablespoons sugar

4 tablespoons baking powder

2 teaspoons salt

12 tablespoons unsalted butter, cold

2 cups whole milk(480 mL)

Method

Preheat oven to 400°F (200°C).

Sift together the flour, sugar, baking powder, and salt in another large mixing bowl. Cut unsalted butter into small chunks and add to bowl or use a cheese grater to grate butter into smaller pieces.

Use a fork to incorporate the butter into the flour mixture until it forms a crumbly texture.

Add milk and stir the dough until it is thick and pulls away from the sides of the bowl.

Transfer dough to a lightly floured, flat surface. Pat the dough down to about 1-inch (2 cm) in thickness, fold in half, and pat down once more to 1-inch (2 cm) in thickness. Cover with a towel and let rest for 30 minutes.

While dough rests, combine chicken, cream cheese, spinach, mozzarella cheese, garlic powder, pepper, and salt in a large mixing bowl.

Lightly flour a rolling pin and roll out dough out to about ½-centimeter (¼ inch) thickness. Use the lip of a cup to cut out 45 circles.

Remove chicken spinach dip from the refrigerator and fill each dough circle with 1 tablespoon of dip. Fold each circle in half and press down the edges to seal the dip inside the dough. Fold the left side and right side of each half circle towards each other like a fortune cookie.

Place the stuffed dough in an 11-inch (28 cm) nonstick or greased tart pan. Make an outer circle and work your way in, creating 4 circles total. Brush with egg wash.

Bake for 25 minutes, or until golden brown.

Enjoy!

Zucchini Carrot Fritters

What You Need -

for 8 fritters

1 cup chickpeas(200 g)

1 zucchini, grated

1 carrot, grated

2 eggs

½ cup whole wheat panko(10 g)

2 teaspoons fresh basil, chopped

½ teaspoon garlic powder

½ teaspoon salt

½ teaspoon pepper

olive oil

GARNISH

plain greek yogurt

green onion, diced

Method

Mash chickpeas with a fork in a large bowl. Set aside.

Grate zucchini. Place in a clean dish towel or cloth.

Grate carrots. Place in a clean dish towel or cloth with zucchini.

Squeeze out as much moisture as possible.

Add veggies, panko, egg, basil, garlic powder, salt, and pepper to the bowl with the mashed chickpeas.

Stir until completely combined.

Heat olive oil in a large skillet on medium heat.

Scoop 2 tablespoons of mixture into your hand press to compress it into a patty.

Cook for about 1-2 minutes, until the underside is golden brown then flip and repeat.

Serve with a dollop of plain greek yogurt and diced green onion.

Enjoy!

The Ultimate Dinner Rolls

What You Need -

for 16 servings

1 cup whole milk(240 mL)

½ cup warm water(120 mL)

¼ cup unsalted butter(60 mL), melted

¼ cup sugar(50 g)

2 ¼ teaspoons active dry yeast, 1 packet

4 cups all-purpose flour(500 g), plus more for dusting

1 ½ teaspoons kosher salt

2 large eggs, room temperature

neutral oil, for greasing

sea salt, for sprinkling

Method

In a liquid measuring cup or small bowl, combine the warm milk, warm water, melted butter, and sugar.

Sprinkle the yeast evenly over the wet ingredients, stir to combine, and let stand for 5 minutes, until foamy

In a large bowl, combine the flour and salt, and stir to combine. Beat 1 egg, then add to the bloomed yeast mixture. Pour the wet What You Need - into the flour and use a knife to stir until the mixture just comes together and forms a dough. Turn the dough out onto a lightly floured surface and knead for 5-10 minutes, or until the dough becomes smooth. Add more flour as needed to keep the dough from sticking. To test if it's done, tear off a small piece of dough and stretch into a thin layer. If the dough doesn't rip, it's ready. Or, press a finger into the dough to see if it bounces back.

Lightly grease a large glass bowl with oil. Add the dough, cover with plastic wrap, and let rest for 1 hour, or until doubled in size.

Punch down the dough, then turn out onto a floured surface. Knead for a few more minutes, just until the dough is smooth, about 2 minutes.

Divide the dough into 16 equal balls, roughly the size of tangerines.

Knead the balls, gathering the edges of the dough toward the center to make a taut, round ball with a smooth top.

Place the rolls on a parchment paper-lined baking sheet. Cover with plastic wrap and let rise for 30 minutes.

Preheat the oven to 375°F (190°C).

Beat the remaining egg in a small bowl. Uncover the rolls and brush with the egg wash. Lightly sprinkle the rolls with sea salt.

Bake for 25-30 minutes, or until the rolls have lightly browned and doubled in size.

Enjoy!

Onion Rings

What You Need -

for 2 servings

nonstick cooking spray, optional

1 large white onion, or large yellow onion

BREADING

1 cup whole wheat breadcrumbs(115 g), or panko bread crumbs (50 g)

½ cup grated parmesan cheese(55 g)

2 teaspoons garlic powder

1 teaspoon paprika

1 teaspoon dried oregano

1 teaspoon dried basil

1 teaspoon salt

½ teaspoon pepper

3 large eggs, beaten

1 cup all-purpose flour(125 g)

dipping sauce, of your choice, optional

Method

Preheat the oven to 425°F (220°C). Grease a baking sheet with nonstick spray or line with parchment paper.

Cut the onion crosswise into ½-inch (1 cm) slices and gently push apart each layer to get individual rings. Set aside.

In a large bowl, combine the bread crumbs, Parmesan, garlic powder, paprika, oregano, basil, salt, and pepper. Add the eggs to a separate large bowl. Add the flour to a third large bowl.

Dredge the onion rings in the flour, then the eggs, then finally in the bread crumb mixture, making sure to coat all sides.

Arrange the onion rings on the baking sheet.

Bake for 10-15 minutes, flipping halfway through, until golden brown on both sides.

Serve with your favorite dipping sauce.

Enjoy!

White Pizza Dip

What You Need -

for 12 knots

pizza dough

8 oz cream cheese(225 g), softened

1 cup shredded mozzarella cheese(100 g)

½ cup grated parmesan cheese(55 g)

½ cup whole milk ricotta cheese(125 g)

¼ cup fresh basil(10 g), chopped

6 cloves garlic, chopped and divided

1 teaspoon red pepper flakes

½ cup butter(115 g), melted

¼ cup fresh parsley(10 g), chopped

Method

Divide pizza dough into 12-14 equal sized balls. With floured hands, roll the dough balls into logs and tie into individual knots, tucking the excess underneath.

Coat a 10 inch (25 cm) oven-safe skillet with olive oil.

Place the knots in a ring around the skillet. Cover with plastic wrap and let rest for 30 minutes, allowing the dough to reach room temperature.

In a medium bowl, combine cream cheese, mozzarella, parmesan, ricotta, fresh basil, 3 cloves of garlic (chopped), and red pepper flakes.

Melt the butter and add the fresh parsley and remaining garlic. Stir well.

Uncover the knots and scoop the dip into the center of the skillet. Brush the knots with the butter/garlic mixture (reserving some for after baking), and top the dip with an additional sprinkle of cheese (optional).

Bake in a preheated oven to 400°F (200°C) for 20 minutes. Broil on high for two additional minutes or until knots and cheese are lightly browned, watching closely so as not to burn it.

Remove from oven and brush lightly with additional garlic butter.

Let cool slightly before serving.

Enjoy!

Loaded Sweet Potato Skins

What You Need -

for 8 servings

4 sweet potatoes

1 tablespoon olive oil

¼ cup whole milk(60 mL)

salt, to taste

pepper, to taste

½ cup shredded mozzarella cheese(50 g)

½ cup shredded cheddar cheese(50 g)

4 strips bacon, cooked until crispy, and crumbled

sour cream, for serving

fresh chive, chopped, for serving

Method

Pierce each sweet potato a few times and bake at 400°F (200°C) for 50 minutes, or until soft.

Let potatoes cool then cut in half lengthwise.

Scoop out potato flesh leaving a thin layer of sweet potato inside, and add flesh to a medium bowl.

Place skins back on baking sheet, drizzle with olive oil and bake at 400°F (200°C) for 10 minutes.

Mash sweet potato flesh with milk, salt, and pepper until smooth and creamy.

Remove sweet potato skins from oven, fill each with an equal amount of potato mixture and top with cheese. Bake at 400°F (200°C) for 15 minutes until the cheese is melted.

Remove skins from oven and top with crumbled bacon. Serve with sour cream and chives.

Enjoy!

Brazilian Chicken Croquettes (Coxinha)

What You Need -

for 9 servings

FILLING

1 tablespoon olive oil

4 cloves garlic, minced

1 white onion, diced

2 cups chicken(250 g), cooked, shredded

½ teaspoon paprika, or cayenne pepper

salt, to taste

4 oz cream cheese(110 g)

3 tablespoons fresh parsley, chopped

DOUGH

1 tablespoon unsalted butter

2 cups whole milk(470 mL)

¼ cup chicken broth(60 mL)

2 cups all-purpose flour(250 g)

egg

2 cups panko breadcrumbs(100 g)

oil, for frying

Method

In a medium pot, heat olive oil, then sauté garlic and onions until soft and brown. Add shredded chicken, salt, and paprika (or cayenne pepper). Stir to incorporate.

Transfer mixture into a bowl, add cream cheese and parsley. Mix well.

In the same pot, add butter, chicken broth, and milk. Bring to a boil. Stir in flour until dough is formed.

Transfer dough to a flat surface. Knead the dough while it is warm, but not hot.

Pinch a piece of dough, about the size of a large egg, and roll into a ball. Using your hands, flatten the dough and spoon filling into the center. Wrap the dough into a pear shape and make sure there aren't any holes.

While heating a pot of oil to 350°F/180°C, dredge the dough in egg and panko, then deep-fry till golden brown and cooked through.

Drain on a towel, or wire rack and serve immediately.

Enjoy!

Chicken Alfredo Bread Boat

What You Need -

for 10 servings

DOUGH

1 cup water(240 mL)

½ cup whole milk(120 mL)

2 ½ cups all-purpose flour(310 g), plus 3 tablespoons, divided

1 tablespoon sugar

1 teaspoon salt

1 tablespoon garlic powder

½ cup grated parmesan cheese(55 g)

1 teaspoon yeast

2 tablespoons olive oil, plus more as needed

CHICKEN ALFREDO

2 ½ cups chicken(310 g), cooked, shredded

2 ½ cups shredded mozzarella cheese(250 g), divided

½ cup grated parmesan cheese(55 g)

1 tablespoon garlic powder

½ teaspoon pepper

2 cups alfredo sauce(520 g)

1 egg, beaten

3 tablespoons fresh parsley, chopped

Method

In a microwave-proof liquid measuring cup, combine the water and the milk. Microwave on high for 45 seconds.

In a large bowl, combine the flour, sugar, salt, garlic powder, Parmesan, and yeast. Mix thoroughly. Pour the milk mixture over the dry ingredients. Stir to combine. Knead the dough on a clean surface for 5 minutes until smooth, if the dough is sticking to the surface add olive oil 1 teaspoon at a time, then form into a tight ball.

Drizzle 2 tablespoons olive oil in a large bowl. Place the dough in the bowl and cover with plastic wrap. Let rise for 1 hour.

Preheat the oven to 450°F (230°C).

In a separate large bowl, combine the chicken, 2 cups (200 g) mozzarella, Parmesan, garlic powder, pepper, and alfredo sauce. Mix thoroughly.

Place the risen dough onto a floured surface. Roll out the dough so it is twice as long as it is wide and about ¼ inch (½ cm) thick.

Transfer the dough to a parchment-lined baking sheet. Roll up all of the sides of the dough to create an oval shape. Pinch the dough and pull it while twisting, wrapping the dough into little spirals and placing it onto the rolled edge of the dough. Continue all the way around until you have several little spirals of dough.

Pour the chicken alfredo mixture over the dough and spread it until it reaches the edges of the dough. Brush the sides of the dough with egg wash. Sprinkle the rest of the mozzarella on top of the chicken alfredo mixture.

Bake for 30 minutes, until the crust is golden brown.

Sprinkle with parsley. Serve immediately.

Enjoy!

Curry Puffs 2 Ways

What You Need -

for 8 servings

1 tablespoon vegetable oil

½ medium white onion, diced

1 ½ lb chicken breast(680 g), cubed

2 teaspoons salt

1 teaspoon black pepper

1 teaspoon ground cumin

2 tablespoons curry powder

½ teaspoon cayenne

2 medium russet potatoes, cooked and diced

1 cup frozen peas(150 g), cooked

1 cup frozen carrot(120 g), cooked

2 cups whole milk(480 mL)

all-purpose flour, for dusting

4 sheets puff pastry, thawed

1 egg, beated, if baking

Method

Preheat the oven to 350°F (180°C), or heat a large pot filled halfway with cooking oil to 350°F (180°C). Place a wire rack on top of a baking sheet.

In large pan, add the vegetable oil, onion, chicken, salt, pepper, cumin, curry powder, and cayenne. Cook for 10 minutes, stirring occasionally, until the onion softens.

Add the potatoes, peas and carrots, and milk and stir to combine. Cook for 10 minutes, stirring to break up the potatoes, until the curry thickens to the consistency of mashed potatoes. Remove the pan from the heat and let the curry cool for 30 minutes.

Dust a clean surface with flour and roll out the puff pastry to flatten the seams.

Using a wine glass, cut out 8 circles from each pastry sheet.

Scoop 1 tablespoon of the cooled curry filling in the center of a puff pastry circle. Fold the puff pastry in half, press the edges together, and seal the edges in a folding and rolling motion.

If baking, place the curry puffs on the prepared baking sheet and brush with the egg wash. Bake for 15 minutes, or until golden brown.

If frying, add the curry puffs to the hot oil in batches and fry for 5 minutes, until golden brown.

Let cool for 10 minutes before serving.

Enjoy!

Pakistani-Style Veggie Pakoras

What You Need -

for 4 servings

2 teaspoons pomegranate seeds, dried

2 teaspoons whole cumin seeds

1 cup chickpea flour(90 g)

1 teaspoon black pepper

1 teaspoon cayenne pepper

1 teaspoon ground coriander

1 teaspoon baking powder

1 teaspoon salt, plus more to taste

2 tablespoons full-fat yogurt

1 cup water(240 mL)

⅓ cup fresh cilantro(15 g), finely chopped

2 small onions, thinly sliced

2 jalapeñoes, seeded and thinly sliced

4 jalapeñoes, whole

3 yukon gold potatoes, peeled and sliced

1 eggplant, peeled and sliced

oil, for frying

mint chutney, for serving

tamarind sauce, for serving

ketchup, for serving

Method

In a mortar and pestle or a spice grinder, crush the pomegranate and cumin seeds, then transfer to a medium bowl.

Add the chickpea flour, black pepper, cayenne, coriander, baking powder, and salt, and stir to combine.

Mix in the yogurt, water, and cilantro, and stir until evenly incorporated. A few lumps are okay. Rest for 15 minutes to let the flour hydrate.

Heat the oil in a large pot until it reaches 350°F (180°C).

Mix the onions and sliced jalapeños into the batter.

Dip the slices of potato, eggplant, and the whole jalapenos into the batter. Try to get the onions and other bits in the batter stuck to the dipped veggies to create more texture.

Fry the dipped vegetables, making sure not to overcrowd the pot, until deep golden brown, about 3-4 minutes.

Drain on a wire rack or paper towels, then salt the pakoras while they are still hot.

Dip in mint chutney, tamarind sauce, and/or ketchup.

Enjoy!

Pizza Popovers

What You Need -

for 6 popovers

3 large eggs

2 large egg whites

1 cup whole milk(240 g), plus 1 tablespoon

2 tablespoons tomato paste

2 teaspoons dried oregano

2 teaspoons garlic powder

2 teaspoons kosher salt

2 ½ tablespoons unsalted butter, melted, divided

1 ¼ cups all purpose flour(155 g)

¼ cup parmesan cheese(30 g), finely grated, plus 1½ tablespoons

½ cup pepperoni(75 g), chopped, divided

1 tablespoon fresh basil, thinly sliced, for garnish

1 cup marinara sauce(260 g), warm

SPECIAL EQUIPMENT

1 6 cup popover pan

Method

Preheat the oven to 425°F (220°C).

In a blender, combine the eggs, egg whites, milk, and tomato paste. Blend until smooth.

Add the oregano, garlic powder, salt, 2 tablespoons of melted butter, and flour and blend on high speed for 2-3 minutes, until completely smooth. Transfer the batter to a liquid measuring cup with a pour spout and let rest at room temperature for 20 minutes.

Meanwhile, place the popover pan in the oven to preheat.

After resting, fold ¼ cup (30 g) Parmesan and ¼ cup (35 g) chopped pepperoni into the popover batter.

Remove the popover pan from the oven and brush ¼ teaspoon melted butter in each cup, then fill ¾ of the way full with batter. Sprinkle with the remaining pepperoni and remaining 1½ tablespoons Parmesan cheese.

Bake the popovers for 25-30 minutes, or until they appear puffed and dry (do not open the oven door to check).

Garnish the popovers with basil and serve immediately with warm marinara sauce alongside.

Enjoy!

Queso Lava Cakes

What You Need -

for 4 servings

QUESO

4 oz cream cheese(115 g), room temperature

4 oz american cheese(115 g), room temperature

4 tablespoons unsalted butter, softened

½ cup shredded monterey jack cheese(50 g)

¼ cup pico de gallo(65 g), drained

LAVA CAKES

nonstick cooking spray, for greasing

1 ¼ cups all purpose flour(155 g), divided

½ cup yellow cornmeal(75 g)

1 tablespoon sugar

½ teaspoon baking powder

1 teaspoon kosher salt

¾ cup whole milk(180 mL)

¼ cup canola oil(60 mL)

1 large egg

2 tablespoons fresh chives, sliced

1 tablespoon chipotle pepper in adobo sauce, drained and diced

FOR GARNISH

½ cup sour cream(120 g)

½ lb chorizo(225 g), cooked

4 fresh cilantro leaves

¼ cup hot sauce(60 mL)

Method

Make the queso: Line a baking sheet with parchment paper.

In a large bowl, combine the cream cheese, processed American cheese, butter, and Monterey Jack cheese and mix with an electric hand mixer on medium speed until smooth and combined. Add the drained pico de gallo and mix with a rubber spatula to incorporate.

Using a ¼ cup measure, scoop out 4 heaping portions of the queso onto the prepared baking sheet. Freeze for at least 2 hours, up to overnight, until completely hardened.

Make the lava cakes: Preheat the oven to 400°F (200°C).

Arrange 4 10-ounce ramekins on a baking sheet. Grease with nonstick spray and dust each with 1 tablespoon of flour, rotating until the ramekins are well coated and tapping out any excess.

In a large bowl, stir together the remaining cup of flour, the cornmeal, sugar, baking powder, salt, milk, canola oil, egg, chives, and chipotles with a rubber spatula until well combined.

Fill each ramekin with 2 tablespoons of the batter and place 1 frozen queso ball in the centers, making sure to keep at least ¼ inch of space between the queso and the sides of the ramekin. Divide the remaining batter between the ramekins.

Bake for 20–25 minutes, until puffed and golden brown on the top. Let cool for 5 minutes before inverting onto plates.

Garnish each lava cake with a dollop of sour cream, chorizo crumbles, a cilantro leaf, and a drizzle of hot sauce, then serve immediately.

Enjoy!

Gravy-Stuffed Cheddar Biscuit Bombs

What You Need -

for 8 servings

SAUSAGE GRAVY

1 lb breakfast sausage(455 g), casings removed

4 tablespoons unsalted butter

¼ cup all purpose flour(30 g)

3 cups whole milk(720 mL)

½ teaspoon dried thyme

¼ teaspoon red pepper flakes

½ teaspoon ground sage

1 teaspoon kosher salt

½ teaspoon freshly ground black pepper

CHEDDAR CHIVE BISCUITS

2 cups all purpose flour(250 g), plus more for dusting

1 tablespoon baking powder

1 stick unsalted butter, cubed

1 cup shredded cheddar cheese(100 g), plus more for dusting

1 teaspoon kosher salt

2 tablespoons fresh chives

¾ cup heavy cream(180 mL)

1 large egg, beaten

Method

Cook the sausage in a large skillet over medium heat for about 5 minutes until evenly browned, breaking up into small pieces as it cooks. Remove from the skillet with a slotted spoon and transfer to a plate, leaving any rendered fat behind.

Add the butter to the skillet. Once the butter melts, add the flour and whisk until light golden brown, about 2 minutes. Slowly whisk in the milk until combined and whisk until the gravy thickens, about 10 minutes.

Add the thyme, red pepper flakes, sage, salt, pepper, and sausage to the pan and stir until combined. Transfer the mixture to a glass measuring cup and let cool to room temperature.

Carefully pour the cooled gravy into a silicone ice mold and freeze overnight.

Make the biscuits: Preheat the oven to 350°F (180°C). Line a baking sheet with parchment paper.

To the bowl of a food processor, add the flour, baking powder, butter, salt, cheddar cheese, and chives. Pulse several times until mixture resembles coarse crumbs.

With the processor running, slowly pour in the heavy cream and pulse until the dough comes together.

Turn the dough out onto a lightly floured surface and knead until no longer sticky. Roll the dough out to about ⅛ inch (½ cm) thick and cut out 8 4-inch (10 cm) circles with a floured biscuit cutter.

Remove the frozen gravy from the mold and place 1 cube at the center of each biscuit. Bring the edges of the dough over the gravy and roll to seal. Save the leftover gravy cubes for another use.

Place the stuffed biscuits on the prepared baking sheet. Brush with the beaten egg and sprinkle with more cheese.

Bake the biscuits for 15–20 minutes, until golden brown.

Enjoy!

Chili Mac 'N' Cheese Pops

What You Need -

for 18 servings

CHILI

1 tablespoon olive oil

1 large yellow onion, diced

1 green bell pepper, diced

1 lb ground beef(455 g)

3 tomatoes, diced

15.5 oz red kidney bean(440 g), 1 can

4.5 oz green chile(125 g), 1 can

3 tablespoons tomato paste

2 teaspoons cumin

½ teaspoon pepper

1 teaspoon salt

1 tablespoon garlic powder

1 tablespoon paprika

¼ teaspoon cayenne pepper

1 lime lime, juiced

ONE POT MAC AND CHEESE

5 cups whole milk(1.2 L)

1 lb elbow macaroni(455 g)

½ cup unsalted butter(115 g), 1 stick

1 teaspoon salt

½ teaspoon pepper

1 ½ cups grated cheddar cheese(165 g)

1 cup grated cheddar cheese(110 g)

9 oz corn tortilla(255 g), 1 bag

1 cup all-purpose flour(125 g)

3 large eggs, beaten

oil, for frying

3 tablespoons fresh cilantro, chopped, for serving

SPECIAL EQUIPMENT

18 bamboo skewers, thick

Method

Heat the olive oil in a large skillet over medium heat, until shimmering. Add the onion and cook until caramelized, about 10 minutes.

Add the green bell pepper and cook until softened, about 3 minutes.

Add the ground beef, break apart, and cook until no longer pink, about 5 minutes.

Add the tomato, kidney beans, green chiles, tomato paste, cumin, pepper, salt, garlic powder, paprika, cayenne pepper, and lime juice. Mix thoroughly and let simmer for about 10 minutes. Remove the pan from the heat and set aside until ready to use.

In a large pot over medium-high heat, add the milk and macaroni. Stir continuously until the milk reaches a simmer and the pasta is cooked.

Turn off the heat, and stir in the butter, salt, pepper, Monterey Jack, and cheddar cheeses. Mix until all of the ingredients are incorporated.

Line a 9x13-inch (23x33 cm) casserole dish with parchment paper so the paper is hanging over the sides of the dish.

Spread a third of the macaroni evenly on to the bottom of the dish and sprinkle half of the cheddar cheese over the top. Spread half of the chili over the cheese. Spread another third of macaroni over the chili, and sprinkle the remaining cup of cheddar cheese on top. Spread the rest of the chili over the cheese. Spread the rest of the macaroni over the chili.

Cover the casserole dish with a piece of parchment paper. Freeze for at least 6 hours, up to 12 hours.

Remove the casserole from the dish using the parchment paper to help you pull it out. Place on a work surface.

Insert 9 skewers into one long side of the casserole 4 inches (10 cm) deep, spacing about 2 inches (5 cm) apart. Repeat on the other long side of the casserole. Cut the casserole in half vertically, then make 8 horizontal cuts in between the skewers.

Crush the corn chips until they are a coarse sand-like texture, then pour onto a large plate. Put the flour and eggs in separate medium dishes.

Place one of the pops in the flour, turning to coat on all sides, and tap off the excess flour. Place the pop in the egg and coat until there is no exposed flour. Place the pop in the crushed corn chips and coat. Repeat with the remaining pops.

Heat the oil in a large pot until the temperature reaches 325°F (165°C).

Fry the skewers 2 at a time for 8 minutes, until browned and crisp.

Transfer to a wire rack or paper towels to drain.

Sprinkle with cilantro and serve immediately.

Enjoy!

Shamrock Empanadas

What You Need -

for 24 empanadas

HORSERADISH HERB SAUCE

2 tablespoons prepared horseradish

¼ cup mayonnaise(60 g)

¼ cup sour cream(60 g)

1 tablespoon fresh chives, chopped

1 tablespoon fresh parsley, minced

½ tablespoon apple cider vinegar

1 teaspoon kosher salt

SPICY MUSTARD SAUCE

½ cup mayonnaise(120 g)

⅓ cup spicy brown mustard(80 g)

1 tablespoon apple cider vinegar

1 tablespoon honey

EMPANADAS

2 qt canola oil(1.8 L), or vegetable oil, for frying

½ lb corned beef(225 g), cooked and cooled

½ cup sauerkraut(75 g), drained

1 cup shredded carrot(50 g)

1 ½ cups cabbage(150 g), steamed, drained and
cooled

¼ cup fresh parsley(10 g), rinsed and stems
removed

1 teaspoon freshly ground black pepper

1 teaspoon ground coriander

1 teaspoon whole mustard seeds

1 teaspoon ground mustard

2 teaspoons kosher salt, plus more for
sprinking, divided

1 cup red potato(140 g), cooled and finely diced

2 large eggs

1 tablespoon water

2 packages empanada dough rounds

SPECIAL EQUIPMENT

clover-shaped cookie cutter, 3 in (7 cm)

Candy or deep fry thermometer

pastry brush

Method

Make the horseradish herb sauce: In a medium bowl, stir together the horseradish, mayonnaise, sour cream, chives, parsley, apple cider vinegar, and salt. Cover with plastic wrap and chill in the refrigerator until ready to serve.

Make the spicy mustard sauce: In a small bowl, stir together the mayonnaise, spicy brown mustard, apple cider vinegar, and honey. Cover with plastic wrap and chill in the refrigerator until ready to serve.

Make the empanadas: Heat the canola oil in a medium pot over medium-high heat until it reaches 350°F (180°C). Set a wire rack over a baking sheet.

In a 4-quart food processor, combine the corned beef, sauerkraut, carrots, cabbage, parsley, pepper, coriander, mustard seeds, ground mustard, and 2 teaspoons salt. Pulse for 30 seconds, until well combined and everything is finely ground. Add the potatoes and pulse for 10–15 seconds more, until the potatoes are very finely chopped but still visible.

Transfer the filling to a sieve set over a bowl and use a rubber spatula to press out any excess liquid.

In a small bowl, beat together the eggs and water.

Lay 2 empanada dough rounds on a clean surface and brush all over with egg wash. Set a 3-inch clover cookie cutter in the center of one of the dough rounds and fill with 1–1½ teaspoons of the filling, mounding in the center of the mold. Remove the cutter and cover the filling with the other dough round, egg wash-side down. Press down firmly with the cookie cutter to seal the filling inside. Using your fingers or a fork, press the edges of the empanada dough together to seal, discarding the dough scraps. Repeat with the remaining dough and filling.

Working in batches of 3–4, gently lower the empanadas into the hot oil and fry for 7–10 minutes, flipping once, until golden brown on both sides. Use a spider to transfer the empanadas to the wire rack and sprinkle with a pinch of salt.

Serve the empanadas hot with the horseradish herb sauce and spicy mustard sauce for dipping.

Enjoy!

Nashville Hot Fried Pickles

What You Need -

for 4 servings

PICKLES

1 ½ lb persian cucumber(700 g), sliced into ½-inch-thick rounds

¼ medium sweet onion, sliced into thin strips

3 pickling salts

3 whole cinnamon sticks, broken in half

3 habanero peppers, slit cut lengthwise down the center of each pepper

1 bunch fresh dill

9 cloves garlic, smashed

2 cups water(480 mL)

¾ cup apple cider vinegar(80 mL)

¾ cup white vinegar(80 mL)

1 cup sugar(200 g)

PICKLING SPICE MIX

½ tablespoon yellow mustard seeds

1 teaspoon brown mustard seeds

2 tablespoons whole black peppercorn

1 tablespoon red pepper flakes

1 teaspoon celery seed

COMEBACK SAUCE

1 cup mayonnaise(240 g)

¼ cup chili sauce(60 g)

2 tablespoons ketchup

1 tablespoon Louisiana-style hot sauce

1 tablespoon lemon juice

1 teaspoon worcestershire sauce

1 teaspoon McCormick® Paprika

1 teaspoon english mustard

½ teaspoon McCormick® Garlic Powder

¼ teaspoon McCormick® freshly ground black pepper

NASHVILLE SPICE MIX

3 tablespoons McCormick® Paprika

2 tablespoons McCormick® cayenne

1 tablespoon McCormick® Garlic Powder

1 tablespoon McCormick® Onion Powder

1 tablespoon McCormick® mustard powder

1 tablespoon McCormick® freshly ground black pepper

FRIED PICKLES

7 cups neutral oil(1.5 L)

1 ½ cups buttermilk(360 mL)

1 tablespoon Louisiana-style hot sauce

2 cups panko breadcrumbs(225 g)

1 tablespoon dark brown sugar

kosher salt, to taste

SPECIAL EQUIPMENT

3 mason jars

deep fry thermometer

Method

In a large bowl, toss the cucumbers and onion with the pickling salt, making sure every piece is well coated. Cover with plastic wrap and refrigerate for 2 hours.

After 2 hours, thoroughly rinse the cucumbers and onion to remove any excess salt. Transfer to a clean large bowl.

Make the pickling spice mix: In a small bowl, mix together the yellow and brown mustard seeds, black peppercorns, red pepper flakes, and celery seeds.

Make the pickles: Scoop 2 tablespoons of the pickling spice mix into each of 3 16-ounce mason jars. Add 2 cinnamon stick halves, 1 habanero, 2 sprigs of dill, and 3 cloves of garlic to each jar. Divide the cucumbers and onion between the jars, packing tightly.

In a small pot, combine the water, apple cider vinegar, white vinegar, and sugar. Bring to a boil over medium-high heat and cook until the sugar has dissolved, 5–7 minutes. Transfer the pickling liquid to a heatproof measuring cup.

Carefully pour the pickling liquid into each jar, leaving ½ inch of headspace at the top. Use the back of a spoon to press down on the cucumbers and onion until completely submerged.

Tightly screw the lids onto the jars and let sit at room temperature for 2 hours, then transfer to the refrigerator overnight, or up to 2 weeks.

Make the comeback sauce: In a medium bowl, whisk together the mayonnaise, chili sauce, ketchup, hot sauce, lemon juice, Worcestershire sauce, paprika, mustard, garlic powder, and black pepper. Cover the bowl with plastic wrap and refrigerate until ready to use, up to 1 week.

Make the Nashville spice mix: In a small bowl, whisk together the paprika, cayenne, garlic powder, onion powder, mustard powder, and black pepper. Transfer to an airtight container and store at room temperature until ready to use. The spice mixture will keep for up to 6 months.

Fry the pickles: In a medium pan fitted with a deep fry thermometer, heat the canola oil over medium-high heat until the temperature reaches 350°F (180°C). Set a wire rack over a baking sheet or paper towels.

Drain the pickles, discarding the pickling liquid and removing any lingering pickling spices, onion, and garlic.

In a shallow dish, whisk together the buttermilk, hot sauce, and 1 tablespoon of the Nashville spice mix.

In a separate shallow dish, stir together the bread crumbs and ½ tablespoon of the Nashville spice mix.

Dip the pickles in the buttermilk mixture, then transfer to the bread crumbs, using your hands to pat the crumbs into each slice until fully coated.

Working in batches, fry the pickles in the hot oil for 3–4 minutes, until golden brown all over. Transfer to the wire rack and season with kosher salt. Reserve 1 cup of the frying oil.

In a medium, heatproof bowl, combine 2 teaspoons of the Nashville spice mix, 1 tablespoon brown sugar, and the reserved frying oil. Whisk until the sugar dissolves.

Brush the hot oil mixture over the fried pickles. Transfer to a platter and serve with the comeback sauce for dipping.

Enjoy!

Pretzels And Beer Cheese Spread

What You Need -

for 6 servings

BEER CHEESE

4 cups shredded cheddar cheese(400 g)

1 clove garlic, grated

1 ½ tablespoons worcestershire sauce

1 ½ teaspoons whole grain mustard

½ teaspoon sweet paprika

¼ teaspoon cayenne pepper, plus more to taste

1 pinch fine sea salt

1 pinch freshly ground black pepper

¾ cup beer(180 mL), ale or lager, at room temperature

PRETZELS

4 cups pretzel stick(512 g)

2 tablespoons unsalted butter

2 ½ teaspoons worcestershire sauce

1 tablespoon white sesame seed

½ teaspoon garlic powder

½ teaspoon onion powder

1 pinch fine sea salt

1 pinch freshly ground black pepper

Method

Preheat oven to 300°F (150°C).

In a large bowl, whisk together the melted butter, Worcestershire sauce, sesame seeds, garlic powder, onion powder, sesame seeds, salt, and black pepper.

Add the pretzels and toss to coat. Transfer to a baking sheet and spread evenly.

Bake until the pretzels are crisp and the seeds golden, stirring often, 10-15 minutes. Set aside to cool completely.

In a food processor combine the cheese, garlic, Worcestershire sauce, mustard, paprika, cayenne pepper, salt, and black pepper, and pulse to combine.

With the processor running, slowly pour in the beer, blending until the mixture is smooth and spreadable. Season with salt, pepper, and cayenne to taste.

Transfer the beer cheese to a serving bowl and cover with plastic wrap. Refrigerate for at least 2 hours or up to overnight.

Serve beer cheese with pretzels.

Enjoy!

Baked Delicata Squash Rings With Honey Mustard Dipping Sauce

What You Need -

for 4 servings

10 oz delicata squash(285 g)

1 cup panko breadcrumbs(50 g), or whole wheat bread crumbs

½ cup parmesan cheese, grated

2 teaspoons garlic powder

1 teaspoon paprika

1 teaspoon dried basil

1 teaspoon dried oregano

1 teaspoon kosher salt

½ teaspoon black pepper

3 large eggs

1 cup all-purpose flour(125 g)

HONEY MUSTARD DIPPING SAUCE

¼ cup dijon mustard(60 g)

1 tablespoon whole grain mustard

1 tablespoon honey

Method

Preheat oven to 425°F (220°C).

Cut 1 inch (2.5 cm) off the top and bottom of each squash, so you reach the seeds. Discard the top and bottom pieces. Slice the remaining squash into ¼-inch (½ cm) thick rounds.

Use a metal teaspoon to scoop out the seeds from the rings.

In a medium bowl, whisk together the bread crumbs, Parmesan, garlic powder, paprika, basil, oregano, salt, and pepper.

In another bowl, beat the eggs. Add the flour to another bowl.

Coat each squash ring in the flour, tapping off any excess. Next, coat in the eggs. Finally, coat in the bread crumb mixture, making sure to press the breadcrumbs into the squash to adhere. Place the coated rings on a baking sheet.

Bake the squash rings for 15-20 minutes, or until golden brown, flipping once halfway through cooking.

Make the honey mustard dipping sauce: In a small bowl, mix together the Dijon, whole-grain mustard, and honey. Use immediately or refrigerate in an airtight container until ready to serve, up to 3 days.

Serve the squash rings with the dipping sauce.

Nutrition Calories: 180 Total fat: 6 grams Sodium: 820 mg Total carbs: 25 grams Dietary fiber: 4 grams Sugars: 4 grams Protein: 9 grams

Enjoy!

Blossoming Onion Lotus

What You Need -

for 6 servings

5 qt vegetable oil(4 L)

2 cups all-purpose flour(250 g)

1 tablespoon garlic powder

1 tablespoon paprika

2 tablespoons pepper

1 tablespoon onion powder

1 tablespoon cayenne

3 tablespoons salt, divided

1 cup whole milk(240 mL)

2 medium russet potatoes

1 large white onion

fresh parsley, for garnish, finely chopped

ketchup, for serving

ranch dressing, for serving

Method

Heat the oil in a 6-quart (5 ½ L) Dutch oven over high heat until it reaches 375°F (190°C).

In a medium bowl, combine flour, garlic powder, paprika, pepper, onion powder, cayenne, and 1 tablespoon of salt and whisk well.

In a liquid measuring cup with a spout, whisk together the milk and half of the flour-spice mix.

Slice the potatoes on a mandolin or with a sharp knife into $\frac{1}{16}$-inch (1 mm) thick slices.

Transfer the potato slices to a large bowl and cover with water. Move the potato slices around to remove excess starch, then drain the water.

Sprinkle the potato slices with the remaining 2 tablespoons of salt and toss to coat.

On a cutting board, slice off the very top and bottom of the onion.

Cut 8 equal slits into the onion, taking care to leave the onion attached at the root end.

Place a potato slice between each onion layer.

Transfer the onion potato lotus onto a spider or fine-mesh strainer.

Place the spider over a medium bowl and drizzle the spice batter over the lotus.

Use your fingers to prod between the layers to ensure the batter soaks into the nooks and crannies of the onion.

Pour the remaining spice mixture over the onion lotus.

Use your fingers to prod between the layers to ensure even coverage.

Fry the onion lotus for 10 minutes, or until golden brown.

Transfer the onion lotus onto a wire rack set over a baking sheet.

Garnish with parsley.

Serve warm, with ketchup and ranch dressing for dipping.

Enjoy!

SECTION 6: FINALLY!

Carcinoid syndrome stands as an incredibly rare medical anomaly, characterized by a spectrum of symptoms ranging from fever, diarrhea, wheezing, to profound fatigue. Despite its enigmatic etiology, the prevailing notion attributes the onset of these manifestations to neuroendocrine tumors. Treatment modalities span from surgical intervention to systemic therapies and symptom-focused medications, contingent upon the size and location of the tumor.

Beyond conventional medical interventions, lifestyle modifications, including dietary adjustments, emerge as pivotal in managing the disease trajectory. Many individuals grappling with Carcinoid Syndrome are able to navigate their daily lives with a semblance of normalcy, aided by a combination of medical regimens and behavioral adaptations.

Notwithstanding its rarity, ongoing scientific endeavors persistently seek to refine treatment strategies and enhance prognostic outcomes for those afflicted with this condition. A robust network of support services and informational reservoirs stands ready to assist patients and their loved ones on their journey towards wellness, underscoring the collective commitment to ameliorating the challenges posed by Carcinoid Syndrome.

To the Reader, From the Author

Carcinoid syndrome is a multifaceted medical condition that exerts a significant impact on an individual's overall quality of life. Although a definitive cure remains elusive, there exist various treatments capable of mitigating symptoms and enhancing the overall quality of life for affected individuals. The effective management of this condition often necessitates a comprehensive, multidisciplinary approach, integrating medical interventions, dietary adjustments, and lifestyle modifications.

Central to the successful management of carcinoid syndrome is the establishment of a robust support network, encompassing not only healthcare professionals but also peers, family members, and advocacy organizations. This network serves as a vital source of emotional support, practical guidance, and access to educational resources. Moreover, advocacy efforts play a pivotal role in raising awareness about the condition and mobilizing support for research endeavors aimed at advancing treatment modalities and improving outcomes for patients grappling with carcinoid syndrome.

By fostering a collaborative environment that encourages dialogue, education, and innovation, the collective efforts of healthcare providers, patients, caregivers, and advocacy groups can contribute to the development of more effective therapeutic strategies and ultimately enhance the well-being of individuals affected by carcinoid syndrome.